Essentials of Audiology

Essentials of Audiology

Felix Priestley

FA
FOSTER
ACADEMICS

www.fosteracademics.com

www.fosteracademics.com

FOSTER ACADEMICS

Cataloging-in-Publication Data

Essentials of audiology / Felix Priestley.
p. cm.
Includes bibliographical references and index.
ISBN 978-1-63242-590-4
1. Audiology. 2. Hearing. 3. Audiology--Instruments. I. Priestley, Felix.
RF290 .E87 2019
617.8--dc23

Foster Academics,
118-35 Queens Blvd., Suite 400,
Forest Hills, NY 11375, USA

ISBN 978-1-63242-590-4 (Hardback)

Printed and bound in China.

Contents

Preface VII

Chapter 1 **Introduction to Hearing** **1**
- Hearing Range 7
- Sound Localization 12
- Auditory Masking 23
- Absolute Threshold of Hearing 32

Chapter 2 **Auditory System** **35**
- Outer Ear 37
- Middle Ear 43
- Inner Ear 50
- Hair Cell 56
- Neuronal Encoding of Sound 61
- Neuronal Structure 68

Chapter 3 **Understanding Audiometry** **91**
- Temporal Envelope and Fine Structure 103
- Auditory Scene Analysis 119
- Audiometer 123
- Sound Level Meter 125
- Noise Dosimeter 135
- Equal-loudness Contour 138
- Noise Map 144
- Noise Measurement 146

Chapter 4 **Hearing Loss and Disorders** **150**
- Hearing Loss 150
- Ménière's Disease 204
- Tinnitus 211
- Hyperacusis 217
- Musical Ear Syndrome 220

Permissions

Index

Preface

Audiology is the science that is concerned with the study of hearing, balance and related disorders. The diagnosis of disorders involves various testing strategies to determine the degree of the loss of hearing, the area affected and the location of the lesion. Testing strategies include otoacoustic emission measurements, hearing tests, videonystagmography and electrophysiologic tests. Cochlear implants, hearing aids, etc. can be recommended depending on the degree of the impairment. This book provides comprehensive insights into the field of audiology. Such selected concepts that redefine this field have been presented herein. Coherent flow of topics, student-friendly language and extensive use of examples make this book an invaluable source of knowledge.

A detailed account of the significant topics covered in this book is provided below:

Chapter 1- Hearing is the ability of humans to perceive sounds through a sensory organ, the ear, by detecting vibrations in the surrounding medium. Some of the topics crucial to the understanding of hearing and sound perception such as hearing range, sound localization, auditory masking and the absolute threshold of hearing have been elaborated in comprehensive detail in this chapter.

Chapter 2- The sensory organs and the auditory parts of the sensory system, whose proper functioning is essential for the sense of hearing or the perception of sound, comprise the auditory system. This chapter has been carefully written to provide an easy understanding of the structure of the auditory system with an emphasis on the outer, middle and inner ear as well as the neuronal structure and the mechanism of the neuronal encoding of sound.

Chapter 3- Audiometry is a branch of audiology that is concerned with the measurement of the hearing acuity relative to variations in pitch, intensity or frequency. The topics elaborated in this chapter, such as temporal envelope and fine structure, auditory scene analysis, sound level meter, noise measurement, etc. will help in providing a better perspective about the basics of audiometry.

Chapter 4- Hearing loss can be of different kinds, such as sensorineural hearing loss, nonsyndronic deafness, unilateral hearing loss, etc. This chapter discusses in detail the different kinds of hearing disorders such as Ménière's disease, tinnitus, hyperacusis and musical ear syndrome.

It gives me an immense pleasure to thank our entire team for their efforts. Finally in the end, I would like to thank my family and colleagues who have been a great source of inspiration and support.

Felix Priestley

1

Introduction to Hearing

Hearing is the ability of humans to perceive sounds through a sensory organ, the ear, by detecting vibrations in the surrounding medium. Some of the topics crucial to the understanding of hearing and sound perception such as hearing range, sound localization, auditory masking and the absolute threshold of hearing have been elaborated in comprehensive detail in this chapter.

Hearing is the ability to perceive sound by detecting vibrations through the ear. Humans have a fairly narrow range of hearing compared to other species – frequencies that we are capable of hearing are between 20 Hz and 20,000 Hz, this is know as the *audio*, or *sonic*, range. Frequencies above that range are know as *ultrasonic* and those below are know as *infrasonic*. Dogs can hear ultrasound, that's why they hear dog whistles and we don't. Apparently snakes can sense infrasound though their bellies, and elephants, giraffes, dolphins and whales use it to communicate.

Listening and hearing are distinction is important, especially when it comes to understanding a hearing loss and successfully using hearing aids. Listening is something you consciously do, it is the act of interpreting and understanding the sound that you heard.

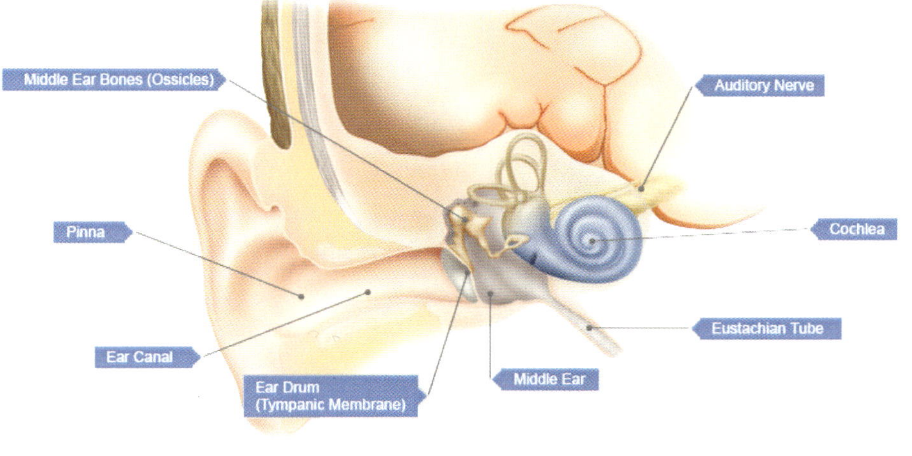

Hearing is an essential part of how we communicate with others and become aware of sounds that happen in our immediate environment. Our hearing abilities start in our ears with the channeling of sound along the hearing pathway which are turned into electrical signs that travel to the brain (shown in the diagram above).

The hearing pathway is divided into four distinct sections that play important and unique parts in our overall hearing abilities.

- Outer Ear
- Middle Ear
- Inner Ear
- Vestibule.

Hearing Loss occurs when one or more parts of the ear or the parts of the brain that make up the hearing pathway do not function normally.

Outer Ear

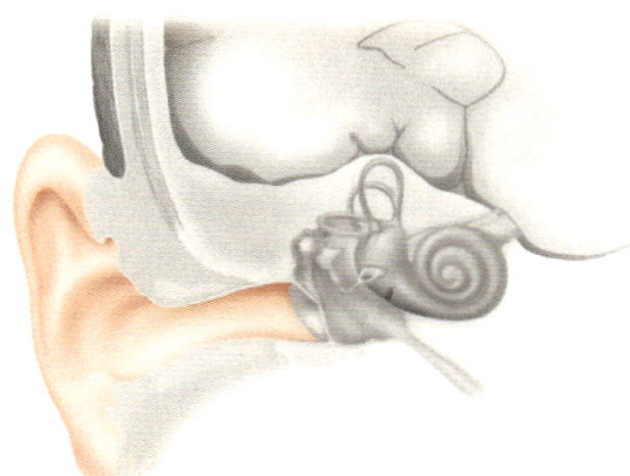

The Outer Ear.

The Outer Ear captures and concentrates the sounds we hear and channels them into the Middle Ear. The Outer Ear is made up of two parts called the Pinna and the Ear Canal. The Pinna is a soft and flexible tissue that makes up the most of the visible ear. It plays an important role in shaping the sound to help the brain work out the direction from which sounds are coming.

The Ear Canal is the physical pathway that directs sound, which has arrived at the Outer Ear, also known as the Pinna into the Middle Ear.

Middle Ear

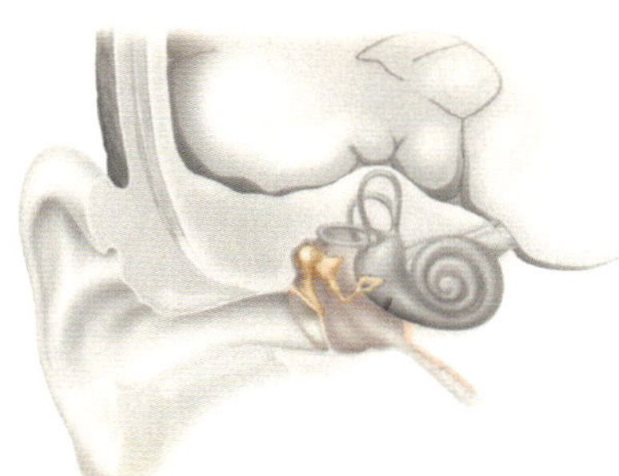

The Middle Ear.

The Middle Ear starts with the Tympanic Membrane, better known as the Eardrum, which vibrates due to differences in pressure caused by soundwaves.

The Eardrum is connected to three small interconnected bones called the Ossicles that vibrate with the Eardrum.

The last of these bones, called the Stapes, the passes on these vibrations into the Inner Ear.

Inner Ear

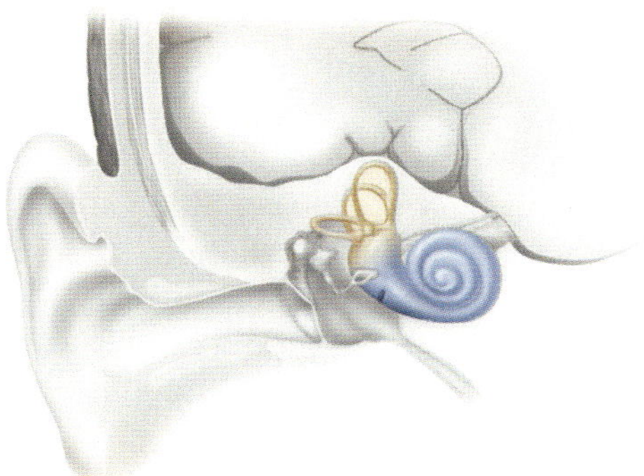

The Inner Ear.

The Inner Ear contains the organs that create our sense of hearing and balance. The Cochlea is the organ in that converts mechanical sound vibrations into nerve signals. using hair-like nerve filaments, called hair cells. These hair cells are arranged so that different cells respond to different pitches.

The electrical currents produced in the Cochlea are then transmitted to the auditory nerve, which passs through several 'relay stations' in the Brainstem before reaching a more complex part of the brain, the Auditory Cortex, where the information contained sound can interpret and understood.

The Vestibule

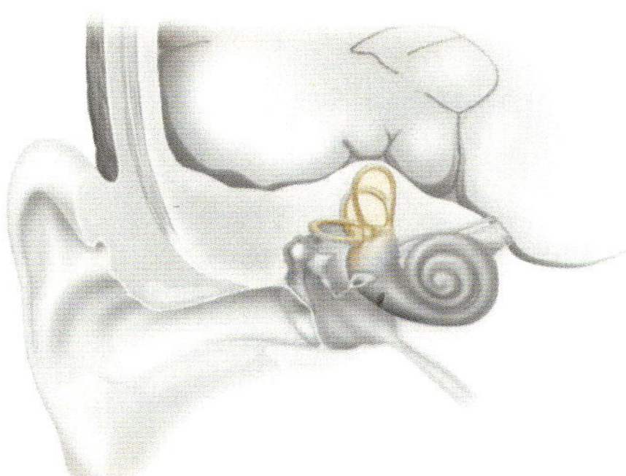

The Vestibule.

The Vestibule, with its Semicircular Canals, is the organ that provides us with our sense of balance, direction and spatial orientation. Vestibule problems can be linked to hearing problems such as Hyperacusis, Meniere's Disease, Tinnitus and Vertigo, which can also affect a person's balance.

Hearing Tests

Hearing can be measured by behavioral tests using an audiometer. Electrophysiological tests of hearing can provide accurate measurements of hearing thresholds even in unconscious subjects. Such tests include auditory brainstem evoked potentials (ABR), otoacoustic emissions (OAE) and electrocochleography (ECochG). Technical advances in these tests have allowed hearing screening for infants to become widespread.

Hearing Loss

There are several different types of hearing loss: Conductive hearing loss, sensorineural hearing loss and mixed types.

- Conductive hearing loss
- Sensorineural hearing loss
- Mixed hearing loss

There are defined degrees of hearing loss:

- Mild hearing loss - People with mild hearing loss have difficulties keeping up with conversations, especially in noisy surroundings. The most quiet sounds that people with mild hearing loss can hear with their better ear are between 25 and 40 dB HL.
- Moderate hearing loss - People with moderate hearing loss have difficulty keeping up with conversations when they are not using a hearing aid. On average, the most quiet sounds heard by people with moderate hearing loss with their better ear are between 40 and 70 dB HL.
- Severe hearing loss - People with severe hearing loss depend on powerful hearing aid. However, they often rely on lip-reading even when they are using hearing aids. The most quiet sounds heard by people with severe hearing loss with their better ear are between 70 and 95 dB HL.
- Profound hearing loss - People with profound hearing loss are very hard of hearing and they mostly rely on lip-reading and sign language. The most quiet sounds heard by people with profound hearing loss with their better ear are from 95 dB HL or more.

Causes

- Heredity
- Congenital conditions
- Presbycusis
- Acquired
  - Noise-induced hearing loss
  - Ototoxic drugs and chemicals
  - Infection

Prevention

Hearing protection is the use of devices designed to prevent Noise-Induced Hearing Loss (NIHL), a type of post-lingual hearing impairment. The various means used to prevent hearing loss generally focus on reducing the levels of noise to which people are exposed. One way this is done is through environmental modifications such as acoustic quieting, which may be achieved with as basic a measure as lining a room with curtains, or as complex a measure as employing an anechoic chamber, which absorbs nearly all sound. Another means is the use of devices such as earplugs, which are inserted into the ear canal to block noise, or earmuffs, objects designed to cover a person's ears entirely.

Management

- Hearing aids are electronic devices that enable a person with hearing loss to receive sounds at certain amplitudes. This technological development has led to the benefit of improving the sense of hearing of a person, but the usage of these devices is significantly low. Psychologically, the first time that a person realizes that he/she needs help from a professional such as an audiologist is when they feel that their hearing is severely poor. Initially, people don't like to believe that they are becoming deaf; hence it negatively affects their approach towards the use of hearing aids. Familiarity with the devices and consultation with professionals do help people feel good about using the hearing aids.

Hearing Underwater

Hearing threshold and the ability to localize sound sources are reduced underwater in humans but not in aquatic animals, including whales, seals, and fishes which have ears adapted to process water borne sound. Some research suggests underwater hearing in humans may occur through bone conduction but with poor localization. This is related to differences of the speed of sound in water vs air and the blocking of normal air conducted sound paths.

Not all sounds are normally audible to all animals. Each species has a range of normal hearing for both amplitude and frequency. Many animals use sound to communicate with each other, and hearing in these species is particularly important for survival and reproduction. In species that use sound as a primary means of communication, hearing is typically most acute for the range of pitches produced in calls and speech.

Frequency Range

Frequencies capable of being heard by humans are called audio or sonic. The range is typically considered to be between 20 Hz and 20,000 Hz. Frequencies higher than audio are referred to as ultrasonic, while frequencies below audio are referred to as infrasonic. Some bats use ultrasound for echolocation while in flight. Dogs are able to hear ultrasound, which is the principle of 'silent' dog whistles. Snakes sense infrasound through their jaws, and baleen whales, giraffes, dolphins and elephants use it for communication. Some fish have the ability to hear more sensitively due to a well-developed, bony connection between the ear and their swim bladder. The "aid to the deaf" of fishes appears in some species such as carp and herring.

Bone Conduction

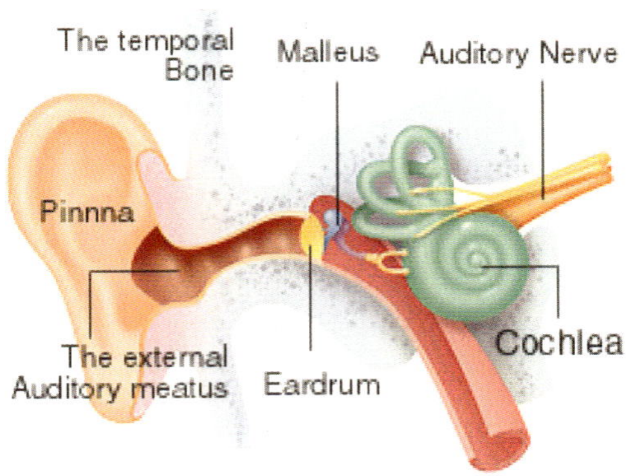

We all hear sounds through both our bones (bone-conducted or bone-transmitted) and our eardrums (air-conducted or air-transmitted). Most sounds are heard by our eardrums. The eardrum converts the sound waves to vibrations and transmits them to the cochlea (or inner ear). However in some cases vibrations are heard directly by the inner ear bypassing your eardrums. In fact, this is one of the ways you hear your own voice. This is also how whales hear.

Normal sound waves are actually tiny vibrations in the air. The vibrations travel through the air to our eardrums. The eardrums in turn vibrate, decoding these sound waves into a different type of vibrations that are received by the Cochlea, also known as the inner ear. The Cochlea is connected to our auditory nerve, which transmits the sounds to our brain.

How we Hear with Bone Conduction

Bone Conduction bypasses the eardrums. In bone conduction listening, the bone conduction devices (such as headphones) perform the role of your eardrums. These devices decode sound waves and convert them into vibrations that can be received directly by the Cochlea so the eardrum is never involved. The "sound" reach the ears as vibrations through the bones (or skull) and skin.

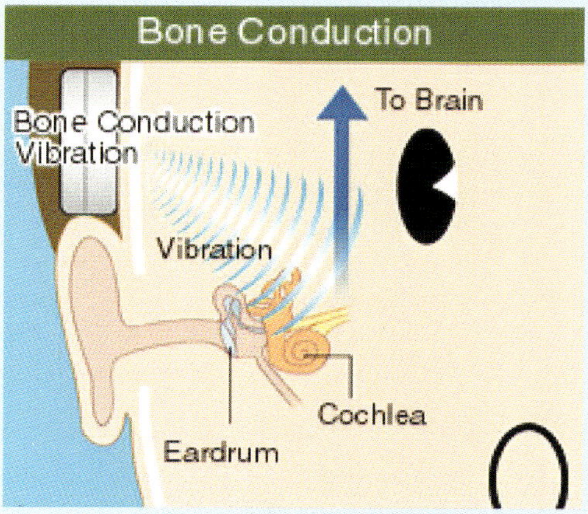

The Basic Idea of Bone conduction is, Bone Vibration makes us hearable.

Most cases of hearing loss are due to damages to the eardrums. Since bone conduction does not use the eardrums, people with hearing difficulties would be able to hear clearly again with bone conduction, provided that their cochlea is in healthy and normal condition. Generally, hearing loss could be described into three categories. That would be conductive hearing loss, perceptive hearing loss and mixed hearing loss. Conductive hearing loss is associated with faulty transmission of sound and is mostly due to damages to the eardrums. Bone conduction is able to aid a conduction hearing loss because a bone conduction device performs the role of the eardrums. Perceptive hearing loss is associated with difficulty in sensing the vibrations by the auditory nerves at the cochlea. Bone conduction is less effective for perceptive hearing loss. As for mixed hearing loss, it is best to suggest a trial in advance to find out whether bone conduction could be an aid to mixed hearing loss because it differs among individual.

Hearing Range

Hearing is one of the five senses of the body. The ears help the body to pick up sound waves and vibrations. Sound travels in waves through the air, the ground, and various other substances. Sound cannot be seen, but it can be felt by vibrations.

The human hearing range is a description of the pitches and loudness levels a person can hear before feeling discomfort.

There are a variety of sounds in our environment, ranging from faint sounds like bird-song and rustling leaves to louder sounds like music, yelling, and industrial noise. This human hearing range is called the audible range.

Loudness and Pitch

The human hearing range depends on both the pitch of the sound – whether it is high or low – and the loudness of the sound. Pitch is measured in Hertz (Hz) and loudness is measured in decibels (dB).

For a person with normal hearing, when it comes to pitch the human hearing range starts low at about 20 Hz. That's about the same as the lowest pedal on a pipe organ. On the other side of the human hearing range, the highest possible frequency heard without discomfort is 20,000Hz. While 20 to 20,000Hz forms the absolute borders of the human hearing range, our hearing is most sensitive in the 2000 - 5000 Hz frequency range.

As far as loudness is concerned, humans can typically hear starting at 0 dB. Sounds that are more than 85dB can be dangerous for your hearing in the case of prolonged exposure.

The difference between the loudest and faintest sounds that humans can hear is about 120 dB, a range of one-million in amplitude. Listeners can detect a *change* in loudness when the signal is altered by about 1 dB (a 12% change in amplitude). In other words, there are only about 120 levels of loudness that can be perceived from the faintest whisper to the loudest thunder. The sensitivity of the ear is amazing; when listening to very weak sounds, the ear drum vibrates less than the diameter of a single molecule.

The perception of loudness relates roughly to the sound power to an exponent of 1/3. For example, if you increase the sound power by a factor of *ten*, listeners will report that the loudness has increased by a factor of about *two* ($10^{1/3} \approx 2$). This is a major problem for eliminating undesirable environmental sounds, for instance, the beefed-up stereo in the next door apartment. Suppose you diligently cover 99% of your wall with a perfect soundproof material, missing only 1% of the surface area due to doors, corners, vents, etc. Even though the sound power has been reduced to only 1% of its former value, the perceived loudness has only dropped to about $0.01^{1/3} \approx 0.2$, or 20%.

The range of human hearing is generally considered to be 20 Hz to 20 kHz, but it is far more sensitive to sounds between 1 kHz and 4 kHz. For example, listeners can detect sounds as low as 0 dB SPL at 3 kHz, but require 40 dB SPL at 100 hertz (an amplitude increase of 100). Listeners can tell that two tones are different if their frequencies differ by more than about 0.3% at 3 kHz. This increases to 3% at 100 hertz. For comparison, adjacent keys on a piano differ by about 6% in frequency.

Softer Louder

Watts/cm²	Decibels SPL	Example sound
10^{-2}	140 dB	Pain
10^{-3}	130 dB	
10^{-4}	120 dB	Discomfort
10^{-5}	110 dB	Jack hammers and rock concerts
10^{-6}	100 dB	
10^{-7}	90 dB	OSHA limit for industrial noise
10^{-8}	80 dB	
10^{-9}	70 dB	
10^{-10}	60 dB	Normal conversation
10^{-11}	50 dB	
10^{-12}	40 dB	Weakest audible at 100 hertz
10^{-13}	30 dB	
10^{-14}	20 dB	Weakest audible at 10kHz
10^{-15}	10 dB	
10^{-16}	0 dB	Weakest audible at 3 kHz
10^{-17}	-10 dB	
10^{-18}	-20 dB	

Figure: Units of sound inyensity.

The primary advantage of having *two* ears is the ability to identify the *direction* of the sound. Human listeners can detect the difference between two sound sources that are placed as little as three degrees apart, about the width of a person at 10 meters. This directional information is obtained in two separate ways. First, frequencies above about 1 kHz are strongly *shadowed* by the head. In other words, the ear nearest the sound receives a stronger signal than the ear on the opposite side of the head. The second clue to directionality is that the ear on the far side of the head hears the sound slightly *later* than the near ear, due to its greater distance from the source. Based on a typical head size (about 22 cm) and the speed of sound (about 340 meters per second), an angular discrimination of three degrees requires a timing precision of about 30 microseconds. Since this timing requires the volley principle, this clue to directionality is predominately used for sounds less than about 1 kHz.

Both these sources of directional information are greatly aided by the ability to turn the head and observe the change in the signals. An interesting sensation occurs when a listener is presented with exactly the same sounds to both ears, such as listening to monaural sound through headphones. The brain concludes that the sound is coming from the center of the listener's head.

While human hearing can determine the *direction* a sound is from, it does poorly in identifying the *distance* to the sound source. This is because there are few clues available in a sound wave that can provide this information. Human hearing weakly perceives that high frequency sounds are nearby, while low frequency sounds are distant.

This is because sound waves dissipate their higher frequencies as they propagate long distances. Echo content is another weak clue to distance, providing a perception of the room size. For example, sounds in a large auditorium will contain echoes at about 100 millisecond intervals, while 10 milliseconds is typical for a small office. Some species have solved this ranging problem by using *active sonar*. For example, bats and dolphins produce clicks and squeaks that reflect from nearby objects. By measuring the interval between transmission and echo, these animals can locate objects with about 1 cm resolution. Experiments have shown that some humans, particularly the blind, can also use active echo localization to a small extent.

Here are some examples of the decibel levels of typical sounds:

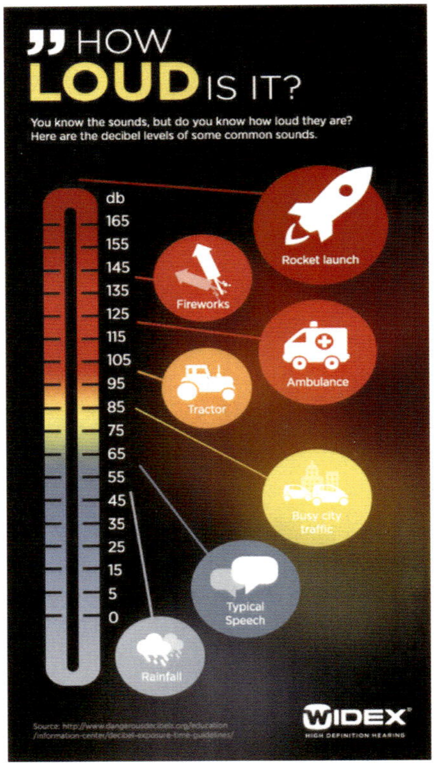

Surprisingly, there are sounds that even humans with the best hearing can't hear. We can't hear the sound of a dog whistle, but a dog can because dogs have a much large hearing range than humans do. Lower frequency sounds like the roar of a wind turbine are also out of the human hearing range and are often felt as vibrations rather than heard as sound.

Hearing Ranges for People with Hearing Loss

When you have a hearing loss, you're hearing range changes. For most, a hearing loss will begin by affecting the upper pitches of the human hearing range. Birdsong, certain speech sounds, and instruments like flutes and piccolos are difficult to hear for most with hearing loss.

To figure out your specific hearing range, a hearing professional will perform a hearing test and plot your results on an audiogram. An audiogram is a chart that shows the results of your hearing test. Your hearing test results are plotted on a graph and then compared with that of a person with normal levels of hearing. Hearing professionals use the audiogram to establish your hearing loss and as a tool for fitting hearing aids.

Here's what an audiogram looks like:

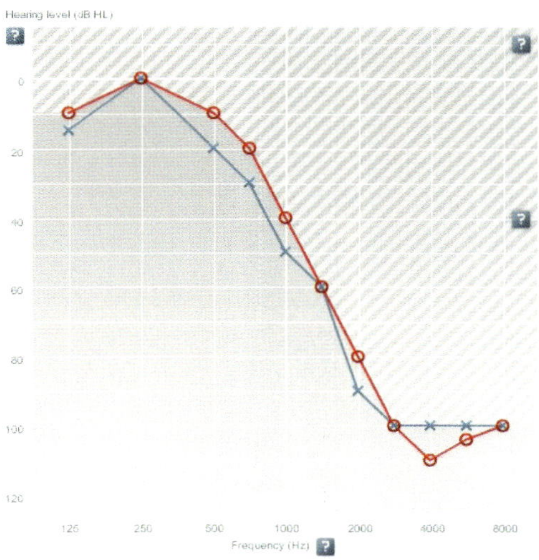

The red line shows the level of hearing of a person's right ear. The left ear is plotted with a blue line. The area below the line shows the levels of hearing loss that this person can hear and the area above the line shows the levels that the person can't hear.

To find out your level of hearing, a hearing professional will play a series of beeps and ask you to raise your hand or press a button when you can hear them. The professional will usually start with a level you can hear and then turn down the volume each time until you can't hear it. The professional will then repeat this with sounds of lower or higher frequencies.

This test shows your hearing "threshold" or the point where you can't hear any more. This threshold is plotted for both your ears as two separate lines on your audiogram.

Your audiogram can tell you a lot about your hearing, including the frequencies you can hear and the volume you can hear them at. This is important to know because each sound you hear has a certain frequency. Birdsong has a higher frequency while tubas have a lower frequency.

Here are some common sounds plotted on a standard audiogram

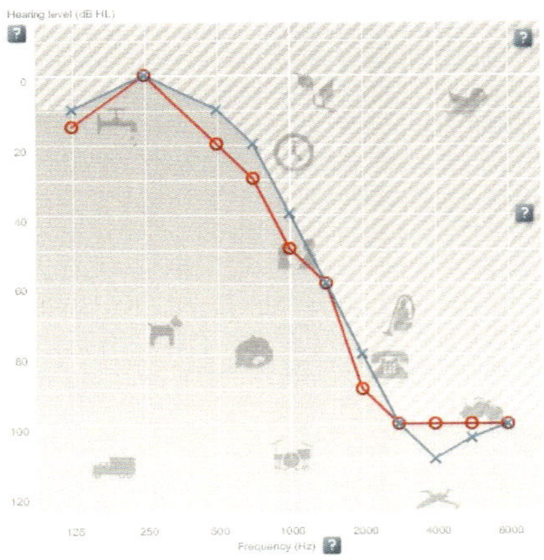

The person with this audiogram has a hearing loss in his left ear that prevents him from hearing sounds like the faucet or birdsong. Lower frequency sounds like the rumbling of a truck engine are easier to hear for the person with this audiogram.

Sound Localization

Sound localization is the ability to tell the direction from which a sound is originating. When sound localization ability is low, it affects a person's safe interaction in an environment. Lack of sound localization ability can influence safe movement in public spaces. If a person cannot tell the direction of an approaching vehicle, with or without accompanying horn or siren, it may lead to fatal consequences.

Sound localization can aid a cat in catching a mouse and can help a person orient to a talker of interest in a crowded party. Beyond just localization, however, normal-hearing listeners can exploit spatial hearing mechanisms to detect and recognize sounds of interest in the presence of other competing sounds. Conversely, people with mild-to-moderate hearing loss report that among their greatest disabilities are the inability to segregate multiple talkers and to understand speech in noisy environments.

Sound localization tasks reflect the extent to which an organism has a well-developed spatial-hearing "map," a perceptual representation of where sounds are located relative to the head. This ability has been studied in adult listeners for decades, with a focus on the extent to which listeners can either identify the exact position of a sound or discriminate changes in the location of sounds. In the former case, localization accuracy has been measured by asking listeners to point to source locations, either by using a pointer object, directing their nose or head in that direction, or labeling source locations using numeric values that refer to angles in the horizontal and vertical dimension.

Accuracy depends on factors such as the task, instructions to listeners, stimulus frequency content and duration, and response options. Error rates are often quantified by the root-mean-square (RMS) error, an estimate of the deviation of responses from the true source location. Results from some studies suggest that RMS errors can be as small as a few degrees.

With children, responses regarding perceived source location are challenging to obtain, and few studies on this topic exist. However, similarly to studies on other aspects of auditory signals, localization prediction has been measured in infants and children using the discrimination paradigm. A common measure is the minimum audible angle (MAA), the smallest change in the angular position of a sound source that can be reliably discriminated. It is important to note that the ability of a listener to discriminate small changes in source location does not automatically generalize to having acute sound localization abilities.

How Sound Reaches the Brain

Sound is the perceptual result of mechanical vibrations traveling through a medium such as air or water. Through the mechanisms of compression and rarefaction, sound waves travel through the air, bounce off the pinna and concha of the exterior ear, and enter the ear canal. The sound waves vibrate the tympanic membrane (ear drum), causing the three bones of the middle ear to vibrate, which then sends the energy through the oval window and into the cochlea where it is changed into a chemical signal by hair cells in the organ of corti, which synapse onto spiral ganglion fibers that travel through the cochlear nerve into the brain.

Neural Interactions

In vertebrates, inter-aural time differences are known to be calculated in the superior olivary nucleus of the brainstem. According to Jeffress, this calculation relies on delay lines: neurons in the superior olive which accept innervation from each ear with different connecting axon lengths. Some cells are more directly connected to one ear than the other, thus they are specific for a particular inter-aural time difference. This theory is equivalent to the mathematical procedure of cross-correlation. However, because Jeffress' theory is unable to account for the precedence effect, in which only the first of multiple identical sounds is used to determine the sounds' location (thus avoiding confusion caused by echoes), it cannot be entirely used to explain the response. Furthermore, a number of recent physiological observations made in the midbrain and brainstem of small mammals have shed considerable doubt on the validity of Jeffress' original ideas.

Neurons sensitive to inter-aural level differences (ILDs) are excited by stimulation of one ear and inhibited by stimulation of the other ear, such that the response magnitude of the cell depends on the relative strengths of the two inputs, which in turn, depends on the sound intensities at the ears.

In the auditory midbrain nucleus, the inferior colliculus (IC), many ILD sensitive neurons have response functions that decline steeply from maximum to zero spikes as a function of ILD. However, there are also many neurons with much more shallow response functions that do not decline to zero spikes.

The Cone of Confusion

Most mammals are adept at resolving the location of a sound source using interaural time differences and interaural level differences. However, no such time or level differences exist for sounds originating along the circumference of circular conical slices, where the cone's axis lies along the line between the two ears.

Consequently, sound waves originating at any point along a given circumference slant height will have ambiguous perceptual coordinates. That is to say, the listener will be incapable of determining whether the sound originated from the back, front, top, bottom or anywhere else along the circumference at the base of a cone at any given distance from the ear. Of course, the importance of these ambiguities are vanishingly small for sound sources very close to or very far away from the subject, but it is these intermediate distances that are most important in terms of fitness.

These ambiguities can be removed by tilting the head, which can introduce a shift in both the amplitude and phase of sound waves arriving at each ear. This translates the vertical orientation of the interaural axis horizontally, thereby leveraging the mechanism of localization on the horizontal plane. Moreover, even with no alternation in the angle of the interaural axis (i.e. without tilting one's head) the hearing system can capitalize on interference patterns generated by pinnae, the torso, and even the temporary re-purposing of a hand as extension of the pinna (e.g., cupping one's hand around the ear).

As with other sensory stimuli, perceptual disambiguation is also accomplished through integration of multiple sensory inputs, especially visual cues. Having localized a sound within the circumference of a circle at some perceived distance, visual cues serve to fix the location of the sound. Moreover, prior knowledge of the location of the sound generating agent will assist in resolving its current location.

Sound Localization by the Human Auditory System

General Introduction

Localization can be described in terms of three-dimensional position: the azimuth or horizontal angle, the elevation or vertical angle, and the distance (for static sounds) or velocity (for moving sounds).

The azimuth of a sound is signaled by the difference in arrival times between the ears, by the relative amplitude of high-frequency sounds (the shadow effect), and by the asymmetrical spectral reflections from various parts of our bodies, including torso, shoulders, and pinnae.

The distance cues are the loss of amplitude, the loss of high frequencies, and the ratio of the direct signal to the reverberated signal.

Depending on where the source is located, our head acts as a barrier to change the timbre, intensity, and spectral qualities of the sound, helping the brain orient where the sound emanated from. These minute differences between the two ears are known as interaural cues.

Lower frequencies, with longer wavelengths, diffract the sound around the head forcing the brain to focus only on the phasing cues from the source.

Helmut Haas discovered that we can discern the sound source despite additional reflections at 10 decibels louder than the original wave front, using the earliest arriving wave front. This principle is known as the Haas effect, a specific version of the precedence effect. Haas measured down to even a 1 millisecond difference in timing between the original sound and reflected sound increased the spaciousness, allowing the brain to discern the true location of the original sound. The nervous system combines all early reflections into a single perceptual whole allowing the brain to process multiple different sounds at once. The nervous system will combine reflections that are within about 35 milliseconds of each other and that have a similar intensity.

Duplex Theory

To determine the lateral input direction (left, front, right), the auditory system analyzes the following ear signal information:

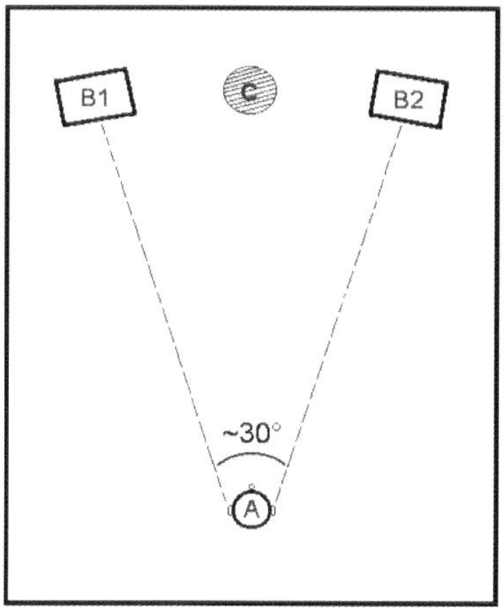

fig. Duplex Theory

In 1907, Lord Rayleigh utilized tuning forks to generate monophonic excitation and studied the lateral sound localization theory on a human head model without auricle.

He first presented the interural clue difference based sound localization theory, which is known as Duplex Theory. Human ears are on the different sides of the head, thus they have different coordinates in space. As shown in figure, since the distances between the acoustic source and ears are different, there are time difference and intensity difference between the sound signals of two ears. We call those kinds of differences as Interaural Time Difference (ITD) and Interaural Intensity Difference (IID) respectively.

ITD and IID

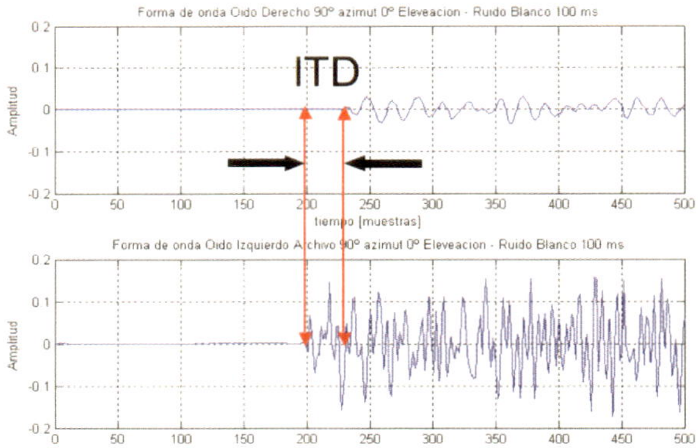

Interaural Time Difference (ITD) between left ear (top) and right ear (bottom).

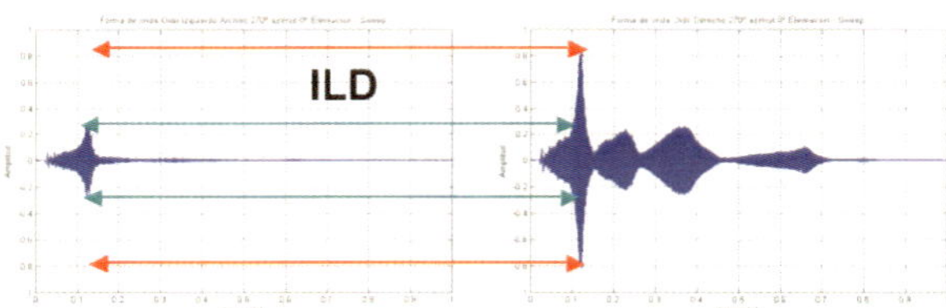

Interaural Level Difference (ILD) between left ear (left) and right ear (right).

From fig. we can see that no matter for source B1 or source B2, there will be a propagation delay between two ears, which will generate the ITD. Simultaneously, human head and ears may have shadowing effect on high frequency signals, which will generate IID.

- Interaural Time Difference (ITD) Sound from the right side reaches the right ear earlier than the left ear. The auditory system evaluates interaural time differences from: (a) Phase delays at low frequencies and (b) group delays at high frequencies.

- Massive experiments demonstrate that ITD relates to the signal frequency f. Suppose the angular position of the acoustic source is θ, the head radius is r and the acoustic velocity is c, the function of ITD is given by: $ITD = \begin{cases} 300 \times \mathrm{r} \times \sin\theta / \mathrm{c}, & \text{if} f \le 4000\text{Hz} \\ 200 \times \mathrm{r} \times \sin\theta / \mathrm{c}, & \text{if} f > 4000\text{Hz} \end{cases}$. In above closed form, we assumed that the 0 degree is in the right ahead of the head and counter-clockwise is positive.

- Interaural Intensity Difference (IID) or Interaural Level Difference (ILD) Sound from the right side has a higher level at the right ear than at the left ear, because the head shadows the left ear. These level differences are highly frequency dependent and they increase with increasing frequency. Massive theoretical researches demonstrate that IID relates to the signal frequency f and the angular position of the acoustic source θ. The function of IID is given by: $IID = 1.0 + (f/1000)^{0.8} \times \sin\theta$
- For frequencies below 1000 Hz, mainly ITDs are evaluated (phase delays), for frequencies above 1500 Hz mainly IIDs are evaluated. Between 1000 Hz and 1500 Hz there is a transition zone, where both mechanisms play a role.
- Localization accuracy is 1 degree for sources in front of the listener and 15 degrees for sources to the sides. Humans can discern interaural time differences of 10 microseconds or less.

Evaluation for Low Frequencies

For frequencies below 800 Hz, the dimensions of the head (ear distance 21.5 cm, corresponding to an interaural time delay of 625 μs) are smaller than the half wavelength of the sound waves. So the auditory system can determine phase delays between both ears without confusion. Interaural level differences are very low in this frequency range, especially below about 200 Hz, so a precise evaluation of the input direction is nearly impossible on the basis of level differences alone. As the frequency drops below 80 Hz it becomes difficult or impossible to use either time difference or level difference to determine a sound's lateral source, because the phase difference between the ears becomes too small for a directional evaluation.

Evaluation for High Frequencies

For frequencies above 1600 Hz the dimensions of the head are greater than the length of the sound waves. An unambiguous determination of the input direction based on interaural phase alone is not possible at these frequencies. However, the interaural level differences become larger, and these level differences are evaluated by the auditory system. Also, group delays between the ears can be evaluated, and is more pronounced at higher frequencies; that is, if there is a sound onset, the delay of this onset between the ears can be used to determine the input direction of the corresponding sound source. This mechanism becomes especially important in reverberant environments. After a sound onset there is a short time frame where the direct sound reaches the ears, but not yet the reflected sound. The auditory system uses this short time frame for evaluating the sound source direction, and keeps this detected direction as long as reflections and reverberation prevent an unambiguous direction estimation. The mechanisms described above cannot be used to differentiate between a sound source ahead of the hearer or behind the hearer; therefore additional cues have to be evaluated.

Pinna Filtering Effect Theory

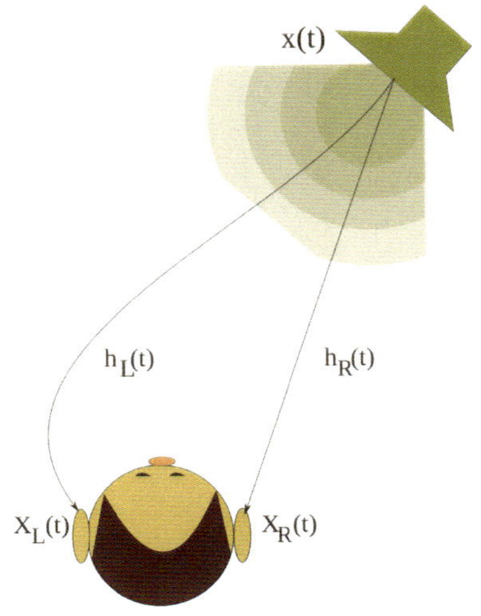

fig. HRTF

Motivations

Duplex theory clearly points out that ITD and IID play significant roles in sound localization but they can only deal with lateral localizing problems. For example, based on duplex theory, if two acoustic sources are symmetrically located on the right front and right back of the human head, they will generate equal ITDs and IIDs, which is called as cone model effect. However, human ears can actually distinguish this set of sources. Besides that, in natural sense of hearing, only one ear, which means no ITD or IID, can distinguish the sources with a high accuracy. Due to the disadvantages of duplex theory, researchers proposed the pinna filtering effect theory. The shape of human pinna is very special. It is concave with complex folds and asymmetrical no matter horizontally or vertically. The reflected waves and the direct waves will generate a frequency spectrum on the eardrum, which is related to the acoustic sources. Then auditory nerves localize the sources by this frequency spectrum. Therefore, a corresponding theory was proposed and called as pinna filtering effect theory.

Math Model

These spectrum clue generated by pinna filtering effect can be presented as Head-Related Transfer Functions (HRTF). The corresponding time domain expressions are called as Head-Related Impulse Response (HRIR). HRTF is also called as the transfer function from the free field to a specific point in the ear canal. We usually recognize HRTFs as LTI systems:

$$H_L = H_L(r,\theta,\varphi,\omega,\alpha) = P_L(r,\theta,\varphi,\omega,\alpha) / P_0(r,\omega)$$

$$H_R = H_R(r,\theta,\varphi,\omega,\alpha) = P_R(r,\theta,\varphi,\omega,\alpha) / P_0(r,\omega),$$

Where, L and R represent the left ear and right ear respectively. P_L and P_R represent the amplitude of sound pressure at entrances of left and right ear canal. P_0 is the amplitude of sound pressure at the center of the head coordinate when listener does not exist. In general, HRTFs H_L and H_R are functions of source angular position θ, elevation angle φ, distance between source and center of the head r, the angular velocity ω and the equivalent dimension of the head α.

HRTF Database

At present, the main institutes that work on measuring HRTF database includes CIPIC International Lab, MIT Media Lab, The Graduate School in Psychoacoustics at the University of Oldenburg, Neurophysiology Lab in University of Wisconsin-Madison and Ames Lab of NASA. They carefully measures the HRIRs from both humans and animals and share the results on Internet for people who want to study.

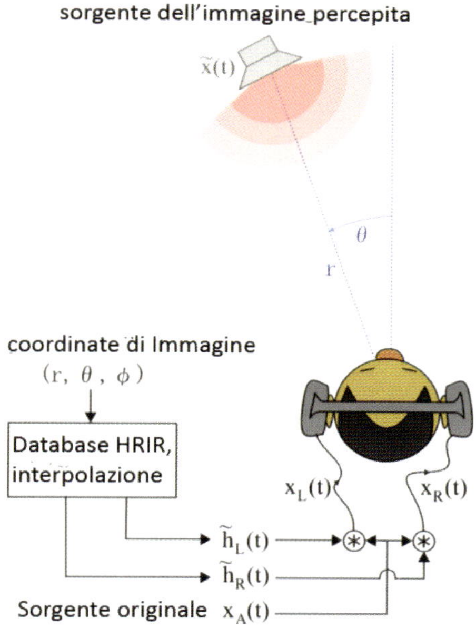

fig. HRIR

Other Cues for 3D Space Localization

Monaural Cues

The human outer ear, i.e. the structures of the pinna and the external ear canal, form direction-selective filters. Depending on the sound input direction in the median plane, different filter resonances become active. These resonances implant direction-specific patterns into the frequency responses of the ears, which can be evaluated by the auditory system (directional bands) for vertical sound localization. Together with other direction-selective reflections at the head, shoulders and torso, they form the outer ear transfer functions. These patterns in the ear's frequency responses are highly individual, depending on the shape and size of the outer ear. If sound is presented through headphones, and has been recorded via another head with different-shaped outer ear surfaces, the directional patterns differ from the listener's own, and problems will appear when trying to evaluate directions in the median plane with these foreign ears. As a consequence, front–back permutations or inside-the-head-localization can appear when listening to dummy head recordings, or otherwise referred to as binaural recordings. It has been shown that human subjects can monaurally localize high frequency sound but not low frequency sound. Binaural localization, however, was possible with lower frequencies. This is likely due to the pinna being small enough to only interact with sound waves of high frequency. It seems that people can only accurately localize the elevation of sounds that are complex and include frequencies above 7,000 Hz, and a pinna must be present.

Dynamic Binaural Cues

When the head is stationary, the binaural cues for lateral sound localization (interaural time difference and interaural level difference) do not give information about the location of a sound in the median plane. Identical ITDs and ILDs can be produced by sounds at eye level or at any elevation, as long as the lateral direction is constant. However, if the head is rotated, the ITD and ILD change dynamically, and those changes are different for sounds at different elevations. For example, if an eye-level sound source is straight ahead and the head turns to the left, the sound becomes louder (and arrives sooner) at the right ear than at the left. But if the sound source is directly overhead, there will be no change in the ITD and ILD as the head turns. Intermediate elevations will produce intermediate degrees of change, and if the presentation of binaural cues to the two ears during head movement is reversed, the sound will be heard behind the listener. Artificially altered a sound's binaural cues during movements of the head. Although the sound was objectively placed at eye level, the dynamic changes to ITD and ILD as the head rotated were those that would be produced if the sound source had been elevated. In this situation, the sound was heard at the synthesized elevation. The fact that the sound sources objectively remained at eye level prevented monaural cues from specifying the elevation, showing that it was the dynamic change in the binaural cues during head movement that allowed the sound to be correctly localized in the vertical dimension. The head movements need not be actively produced; accurate vertical localization occurred in a similar setup when the head rotation was produced passively, by seating the blindfolded subject in a rotating chair. As long as the dynamic changes in binaural cues accompanied a perceived head rotation, the synthesized elevation was perceived.

Distance of the Sound Source

The human auditory system has only limited possibilities to determine the distance of a sound source. In the close-up-range there are some indications for distance determination, such as extreme level differences (e.g. when whispering into one ear) or specific pinna (the visible part of the ear) resonances in the close-up range.

The auditory system uses these clues to estimate the distance to a sound source:

- Direct/ Reflection ratio: In enclosed rooms, two types of sound are arriving at a listener: The direct sound arrives at the listener's ears without being reflected at a wall. Reflected sound has been reflected at least one time at a wall before arriving at the listener. The ratio between direct sound and reflected sound can give an indication about the distance of the sound source.
- Loudness: Distant sound sources have a lower loudness than close ones. This aspect can be evaluated especially for well-known sound sources.
- Sound spectrum : High frequencies are more quickly damped by the air than low frequencies. Therefore, a distant sound source sounds more muffled than a close one, because the high frequencies are attenuated. For sound with a known spectrum (e.g. speech) the distance can be estimated roughly with the help of the perceived sound.
- ITDG: The Initial Time Delay Gap describes the time difference between arrival of the direct wave and first strong reflection at the listener. Nearby sources create a relatively large ITDG, with the first reflections having a longer path to take, possibly many times longer. When the source is far away, the direct and the reflected sound waves have similar path lengths.
- Movement: Similar to the visual system there is also the phenomenon of motion parallax in acoustical perception. For a moving listener nearby sound sources are passing faster than distant sound sources.
- Level Difference: Very close sound sources cause a different level between the ears.

Signal Processing

Sound processing of the human auditory system is performed in so-called critical bands. The hearing range is segmented into 24 critical bands, each with a width of 1 Bark or 100 Mel. For a directional analysis the signals inside the critical band are analyzed together.

The auditory system can extract the sound of a desired sound source out of interfering noise. This allows the listener to concentrate on only one speaker if other speakers are also talking (the cocktail party effect). With the help of the cocktail party effect sound from interfering directions is perceived attenuated compared to the sound from the desired direction. The auditory system can increase the signal-to-noise ratio by up to 15 dB, which means that interfering sound is perceived to be attenuated to half (or less) of its actual loudness.

Localization in Enclosed Rooms

In enclosed rooms not only the direct sound from a sound source is arriving at the listener's ears, but also sound which has been reflected at the walls. The auditory system analyses only the direct sound, which is arriving first, for sound localization, but not the reflected sound, which is arriving later (law of the first wave front). So sound localization remains possible even in an echoic environment. This echo cancellation occurs in the Dorsal Nucleus of the Lateral Lemniscus (DNLL).

In order to determine the time periods, where the direct sound prevails and which can be used for directional evaluation, the auditory system analyzes loudness changes in different critical bands and also the stability of the perceived direction. If there is a strong attack of the loudness in several critical bands and if the perceived direction is stable, this attack is in all probability caused by the direct sound of a sound source, which is entering newly or which is changing its signal characteristics. This short time period is used by the auditory system for directional and loudness analysis of this sound. When reflections arrive a little bit later, they do not enhance the loudness inside the critical bands in such a strong way, but the directional cues become unstable, because there is a mix of sound of several reflection directions. As a result, no new directional analysis is triggered by the auditory system.

This first detected direction from the direct sound is taken as the found sound source direction, until other strong loudness attacks, combined with stable directional information, indicate that a new directional analysis is possible.

Specific Techniques with Applications

Auditory Transmission Stereo System

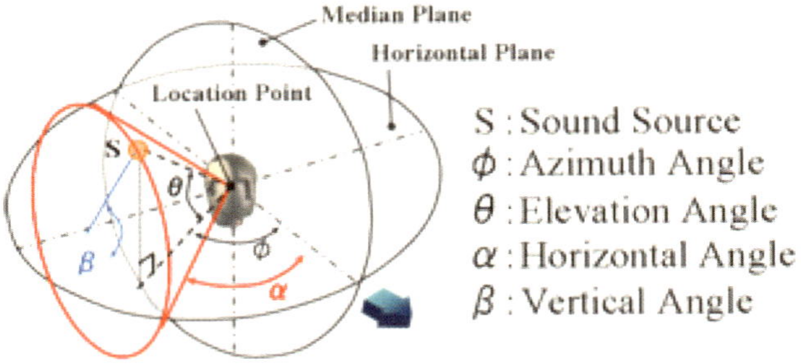

fig: Sound Localization with Manikin

This kind of sound localization technique provides us the real virtual stereo system. It utilizes "smart" manikins, such as KEMAR, to glean signals or use DSP methods to simulate the transmission process from sources to ears. After amplifying, recording and transmitting, the two channels of received signals will be reproduced through earphones or speakers. This localization approach uses electroacoustic methods to obtain the spatial information of the original sound field by transferring the listener's auditory apparatus to the original sound field. The most considerable advantages of it would be that its acoustic images are lively and natural. Also, it only needs two independent transmitted signal to reproduce the acoustic image of a 3D system.

3D Para-virtualization Stereo System

The representatives of this kind of system are SRS Audio Sandbox, Spatializer Audio Lab and Qsound Qxpander. They use HRTF to simulate the received acoustic signals at the ears from different directions with common binary-channel stereo reproduction. Therefore, they can simulate reflected sound waves and improve subjective sense of space and envelopment. Since they are para-virtualization stereo systems, the major goal of them is to simulate stereo sound information. Traditional stereo systems use sensors that are quite different from human ears. Although those sensors can receive the acoustic information from different directions, they do not have the same frequency response of human auditory system. Therefore, when binary-channel mode is applied, human auditory systems still cannot feel the 3D sound effect field. However, the 3D Para-virtualization stereo system overcome such disadvantages. It uses HRTF principles to glean acoustic information from the original sound field then produce a lively 3D sound field through common earphones or speakers.

Multichannel Stereo Virtual Reproduction

Since the multichannel stereo systems require lots of reproduction channels, some researchers adopted the HRTF simulation technologies to reduce the number of reproduction channels. They use only two speakers to simulate multiple speakers in a multichannel system. This process is called as virtual reproduction. Essentially, such approach uses both interaural difference principle and pinna filtering effect theory. Unfortunately, this kind of approach cannot perfectly substitute the traditional multichannel stereo system, such as 5.1 surround sound system. That is because when the listening zone is relatively larger, simulation reproduction through HRTFs may cause invert acoustic images at symmetric positions.

Auditory Masking

It is rare to hear just one sound at a time. More often than not, our experience of listening to someone speak, or hearing a piece of music, is made more challenging, and possibly more annoying, by the presence of interfering sound, be it traffic noise, air-conditioning rumble, or other people talking at the same time. In extreme situations, such as in a noisy restaurant or bar, the background noise may prevent us from even hearing the conversation we are trying our best to follow. This phenomenon is known as masking, and it occurs in every sensory system.

When multiple sound sources are present at the same time, the variations in air pressure produced by each source combine to form a single pattern of rapidly varying air pressure at each of the listener's eardrums, causing them to vibrate. The auditory system must then decompose the patterns of vibrations at the eardrums to provide us with information about the individual sound sources, such as their identity and location. Given this daunting challenge, the question might be how we are ever able to hear out sounds from a mixture, rather than why our ability to do so sometimes fails. A crucial first step in this decomposition process is accomplished within the cochlea, where different frequencies within a complex sound maximally stimulate different places along the length of the basilar membrane – a structure that runs the length of the cochlea. This frequency-to-place mapping, or tonotopic organization, is a fundamental organizational principle of auditory coding and is maintained throughout lower structures of the auditory system, up to and including primary auditory cortex.

Masking tends to occur when the tonotopic representation of one sound interferes with that of another. The 'classical' masking studies in both physiological and perceptual (behavioural) experiments have involved embedding a tonal signal in a noise masker. Physiological correlates of masking have been identified at various levels of the auditory system beginning in the auditory nerve.

Many of the non-linear neural phenomena produced by the interaction of tones and noise, such as frequency-specific suppression of tones by noise (and vice versa), have their origins in the mechanical response of the basilar membrane. In addition, some of the more linear aspects of auditory processing, such as the constant signal-to-noise ratio at threshold over a large dynamic range, provide an early physiological correlate of the perceptual invariance we experience when listening to the same sound over a wide range of stimulus levels.

Masked Threshold

The *unmasked threshold* is the quietest level of the signal which can be perceived without a masking signal present. The *masked threshold* is the quietest level of the signal perceived when combined with a specific masking noise. The amount of masking is the difference between the masked and unmasked thresholds.

Gelfand provides a basic example. Let us say that for a given individual, the sound of a cat scratching a post in an otherwise quiet environment is first audible at a level of 10 dB SPL. However, in the presence of a masking noise (for example, a vacuum cleaner that is running simultaneously) that same individual cannot detect the sound of the cat scratching unless the level of the scratching sound is at least 26 dB SPL. We would say that the unmasked threshold for that individual for the target sound (i.e., the cat scratching) is 10 dB SPL, while the masked threshold is 26 dB SPL. The amount of masking is simply the difference between these two thresholds: 16 dB.

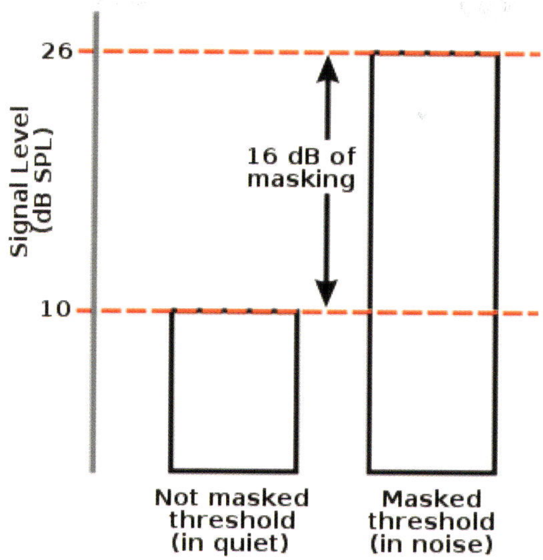

Figure – adapted from Gelfand

The amount of masking will vary depending on the characteristics of both the target signal and the masker, and will also be specific to an individual listener. While the person in the example above was able to detect the cat scratching at 26 dB SPL, another person may not be able to hear the cat scratching while the vacuum was on until the sound level of the cat scratching was increased to 30 dB SPL (thereby making the amount of masking for the second listener 20 dB).

Simultaneous Masking

Simultaneous masking occurs when a sound is made inaudible by a noise or unwanted sound of the same duration as the original sound. For example, a powerful spike at 1 kHz will tend to mask out a lower-level tone at 1.1 kHz. Also, two sine tones at 440 and 450 Hz can be perceived clearly when separated. They cannot be perceived clearly when presented simultaneously.

Critical Bandwidth

If two sounds of two different frequencies are played at the same time, two separate sounds can often be heard rather than a combination tone. The ability to hear frequencies separately is known as *frequency resolution* or *frequency selectivity*. When signals are perceived as a combination tone, they are said to reside in the same *critical bandwidth*. This effect is thought to occur due to filtering within the cochlea, the hearing organ in the inner ear. A complex sound is split into different frequency components and these components cause a peak in the pattern of vibration at a specific place on the cilia inside the basilar membrane within the cochlea. These components are then coded independently on the auditory nerve which transmits sound information to the brain. This individual coding only occurs if the frequency components are different enough in frequency, otherwise they are in the same critical band and are coded at the same place and are perceived as one sound instead of two.

The filters that distinguish one sound from another are called auditory filters, listening channels or critical bandwidths. Frequency resolution occurs on the basilar membrane due to the listener choosing a filter which is centered over the frequency they expect to hear, the signal frequency. A sharply tuned filter has good frequency resolution as it allows the center frequencies through but not other frequencies (Pickles 1982). Damage to the cochlea and the outer hair cells in the cochlea can impair the ability to tell sounds apart (Moore 1986). This explains why someone with a hearing loss due to cochlea damage would have more difficulty than a normal hearing person in distinguishing between different consonants in speech.

Masking illustrates the limits of frequency selectivity. If a signal is masked by a masker with a different frequency to the signal, then the auditory system was unable to distinguish between the two frequencies. By experimenting with conditions where one sound can mask a previously heard signal, the frequency selectivity of the auditory system can be tested.

Similar Frequencies

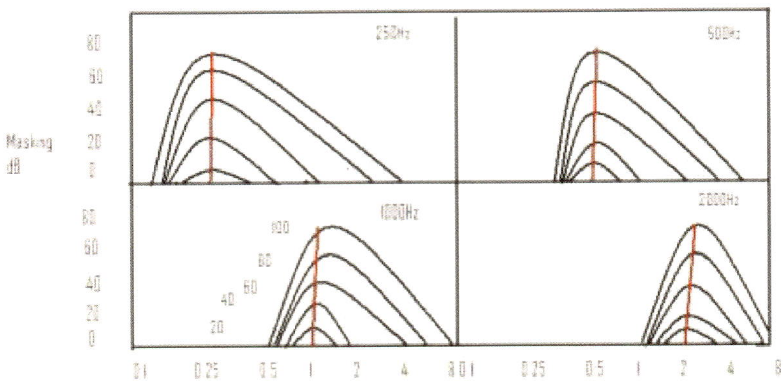

Figure – Adapted from Ehmer

How effective the masker is at raising the threshold of the signal depends on the frequency of the signal and the frequency of the masker. The graphs in figure are a series of masking patterns, also known as masking audiograms. Each graph shows the amount of masking produced at each masker frequency shown at the top corner, 250, 500, 1000 and 2000 Hz. For example, in the first graph the masker is presented at a frequency of 250 Hz at the same time as the signal. The amount the masker increases the threshold of the signal is plotted and this is repeated for different signal frequencies, shown on the X axis. The frequency of the masker is kept constant. The masking effect is shown in each graph at various masker sound levels.

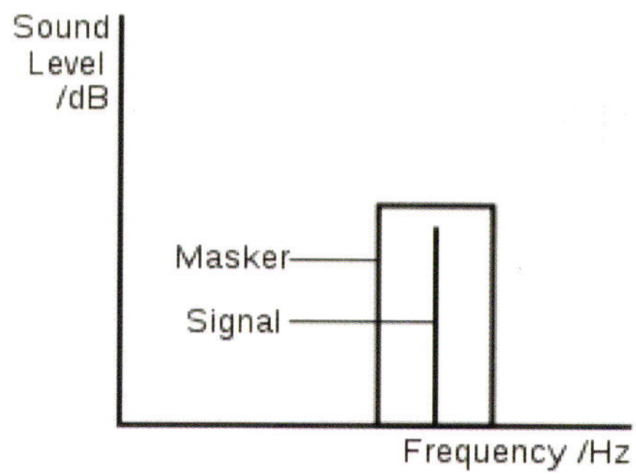

Figure – Adapted from Gelfand

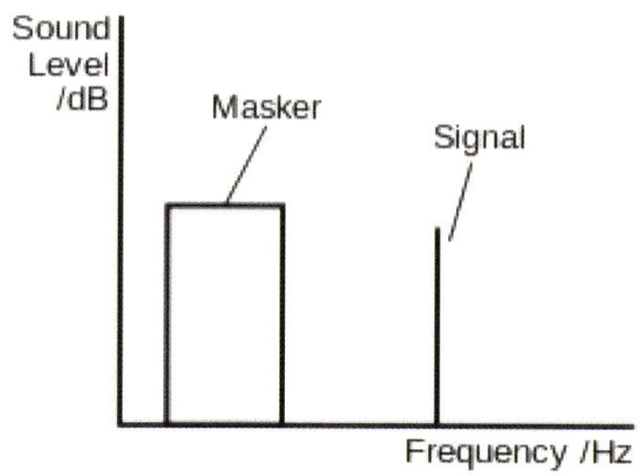

Figure – Adapted from Gelfand

Figure shows along the Y axis the amount of masking. The greatest masking is when the masker and the signal are the same frequency and this decreases as the signal frequency moves further away from the masker frequency. This phenomenon is called on-frequency masking and occurs because the masker and signal are within the same auditory filter. This means that the listener cannot distinguish between them and they are perceived as one sound with the quieter sound masked by the louder one.

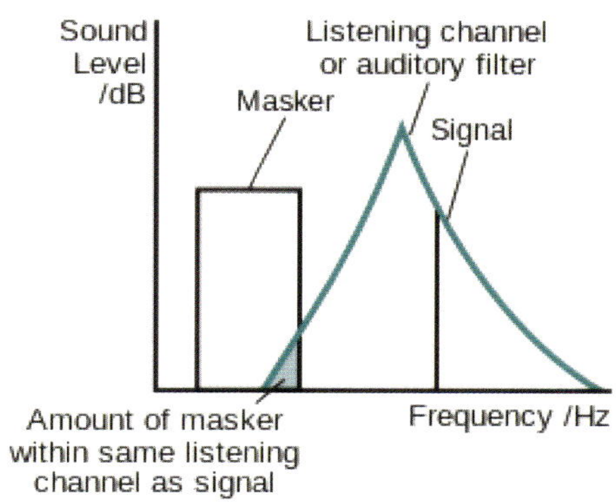

Figure – adapted from Moore

The amount the masker raises the threshold of the signal is much less in off-frequency masking, but it does have some masking effect because some of the masker overlaps into the auditory filter of the signal.

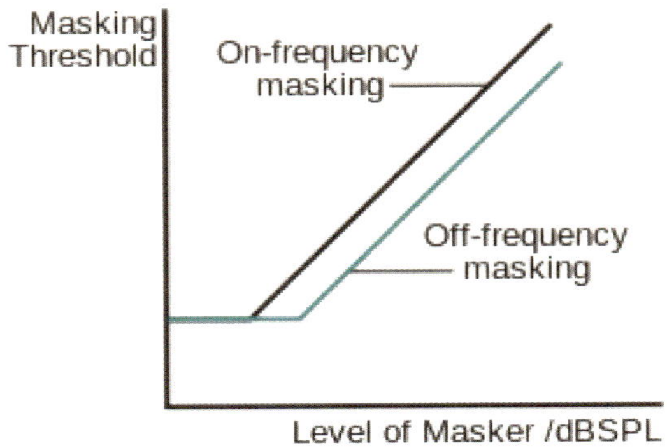

Figure – adapted from Moore

Off-frequency masking requires the level of the masker to be greater in order to have a masking effect; this is shown in figure. This is because only a certain amount of the masker overlaps into the auditory filter of the signal and more masker is needed to cover the signal.

Lower Frequencies

The masking pattern changes depending on the frequency of the masker and the intensity. For low levels on the 1000 Hz graph, such as the 20-40 dB range, the curve is relatively parallel. As the masker intensity increases the curves separate, especially for signals at a frequency higher than the masker. This shows that there is a spread of the masking effect upward in frequency as the intensity of the masker is increased. The curve is much shallower in the high frequencies than in the low frequencies. This flattening is called upward spread of masking and is why an interfering sound masks high frequency signals much better than low frequency signals.

Figure also shows that as the masker frequency increases, the masking patterns become increasingly compressed. This demonstrates that high frequency maskers are only effective over a narrow range of frequencies, close to the masker frequency. Low frequency maskers on the other hand are effective over a wide frequency range.

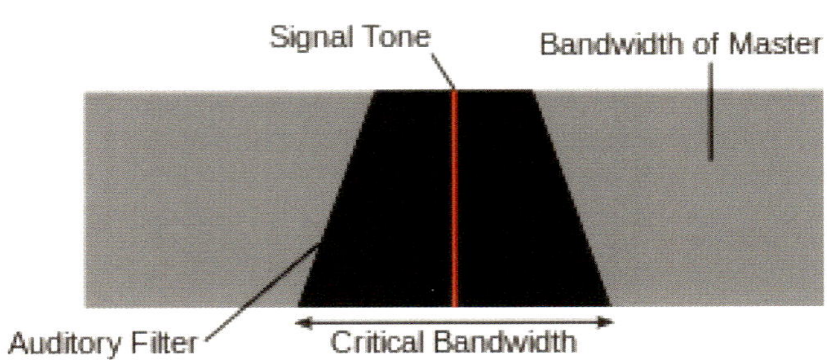

Figure – adapted from a diagram by Gelfand

Harvey Fletcher carried out an experiment to discover how much of a band of noise contributes to the masking of a tone. In the experiment, a fixed tone signal had various bandwidths of noise centered on it. The masked threshold was recorded for each bandwidth. His research showed that there is a critical bandwidth of noise which causes the maximum masking effect and energy outside that band does not affect the masking. This can be explained by the auditory system having an auditory filter which is centered over the frequency of the tone. The bandwidth of the masker that is within this auditory filter effectively masks the tone but the masker outside of the filter has no effect.

This is used in MP3 files to reduce the size of audio files. Parts of the signals which are outside the critical bandwidth are represented with reduced precision. The parts of the signals which are perceived by the listener are reproduced with higher fidelity.

Effects of Intensity

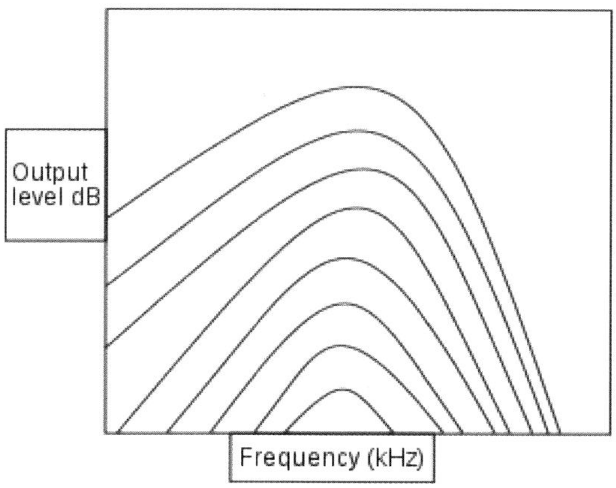

Figure – adapted from Moore

Varying intensity levels can also have an effect on masking. The lower end of the filter becomes flatter with increasing decibel level, whereas the higher end becomes slightly steeper. Changes in slope of the high frequency side of the filter with intensity are less consistent than they are at low frequencies. At the medium frequencies (1–4 kHz) the slope increases as intensity increases, but at the low frequencies there is no clear inclination with level and the filters at high center frequencies show a small decrease in slope with increasing level. The sharpness of the filter depends on the input level and not the output level to the filter. The lower side of the auditory filter also broadens with increasing level. These observations are illustrated in Figure.

Temporal Masking

Temporal masking or non-simultaneous masking occurs when a sudden stimulus sound makes inaudible other sounds which are present immediately preceding or following the stimulus. Masking which obscures a sound immediately preceding the masker is called *backward masking* or *pre-masking* and masking which obscures a sound immediately following the masker is called *forward masking* or *post-masking*. Temporal masking's effectiveness attenuates exponentially from the onset and offset of the masker, with the onset attenuation lasting approximately 20 ms and the offset attenuation lasting approximately 100 ms.

Similar to simultaneous masking, temporal masking reveals the frequency analysis performed by the auditory system; forward masking thresholds for complex harmonic tones (e.g., a sawtooth probe with a fundamental frequency of 500 Hz) exhibit threshold peaks (i.e., high masking levels) for frequency bands centered on the first several harmonics. In fact, auditory bandwidths measured from forward masking thresholds are narrower and more accurate than those measured using simultaneous masking.

Temporal masking should not be confused with the ear's acoustic reflex, an involuntary response in the middle ear that is activated to protect the ear's delicate structures from loud sounds.

Other Masking Conditions

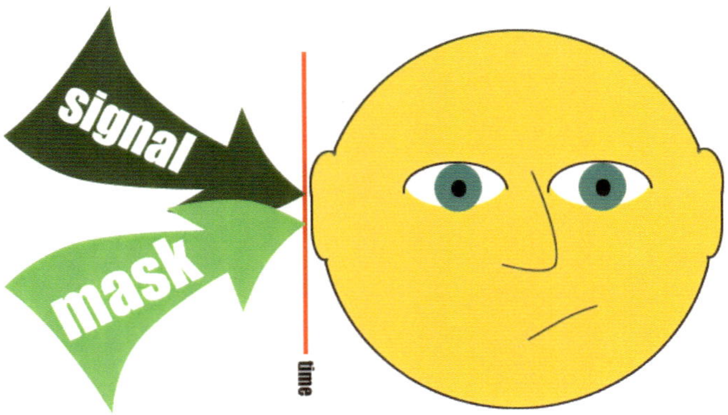

figure – ipsilateral simultaneous masking

Ipsilateral ("same side") masking is not the only condition where masking takes place. Another situation where masking occurs is called contralateral ("other side") simultaneous masking. In this case, the instance where the signal might be audible in one ear but is deliberately taken away by applying a masker to the other ear.

The last situation where masking occurs is called central masking. This refers to the case where a masker causes a threshold elevation. This can be in the absence of, or in addition to, another effect and is due to interactions within the central nervous system between the separate neural inputs obtained from the masker and the signal.

Effects of Different Stimulus Types

Experiments have been carried out to see the different masking effects when using a masker which is either in the form of a narrow band noise or a sinusoidal tone.

When a sinusoidal signal and a sinusoidal masker (tone) are presented simultaneously the envelope of the combined stimulus fluctuates in a regular pattern described as beats. The fluctuations occur at a rate defined by the difference between the frequencies of the two sounds. If the frequency difference is small then the sound is perceived as a periodic change in the loudness of a single tone. If the beats are fast then this can be described as a sensation of roughness. When there is a large frequency separation, the two components are heard as separate tones without roughness or beats. Beats can be a cue to the presence of a signal even when the signal itself is not audible. The influence of beats can be reduced by using a narrowband noise rather than a sinusoidal tone for either signal or masker.

Mechanisms of Masking

There are many different mechanisms of masking, one being suppression. This is when there is a reduction of a response to a signal due to the presence of another. This happens because the original neural activity caused by the first signal is reduced by the neural activity of the other sound.

Combination tones are products of a signal and a masker. This happens when the two sounds interact causing new sound, which can be more audible than the original signal. This is caused by the non linear distortion that happens in the ear. For example, the combination tone of two maskers can be a better masker than the two original maskers alone.

The sounds interact in many ways depending on the difference in frequency between the two sounds. The most important two are cubic difference tones and quadratic difference tones.

Cubic difference tones are calculated by the sum:

$$2F1 - F2$$

(F1 being the first frequency, F2 the second) These are audible most of the time and especially when the level of the original tone is low. Hence they have a greater effect on psychoacoustic tuning curves than quadratic difference tones.

Quadratic difference tones are the result of:

$$F2 - F1$$

This happens at relatively high levels hence have a lesser effect on psychoacoustic tuning curves.

Combination tones can interact with primary tones resulting in secondary combination tones due to being like their original primary tones in nature, stimulus like. An example of this is:

$$3F1 - 2F2$$

Secondary combination tones are again similar to the combination tones of the primary tone.

Off Frequency Listening

Off frequency listening is when a listener chooses a filter just lower than the signal frequency to improve their auditory performance. This "off frequency" filter reduces the level of the masker more than the signal at the output level of the filter, which means they can hear the signal more clearly hence causing an improvement of auditory performance.

Applications

Auditory masking is used in tinnitus maskers to suppress annoying ringing, hissing, or buzzing or tinnitus often associated with hearing loss. It is also used in various kinds of audiometry, including pure tone audiometry, and the standard hearing test to test each ear unilaterally and to test speech recognition in the presence of partially masking noise.

Auditory masking is exploited to perform data compression for sound signals (MP3).

Absolute Threshold of Hearing

The human ear has incredible absolute sensitivity and dynamic range. The most intense sound we can hear without immediate damage to the ear is at least 140 dB above the faintest sound we can just detect. This corresponds to an intensity ratio of 100 000 000 000 000:1.

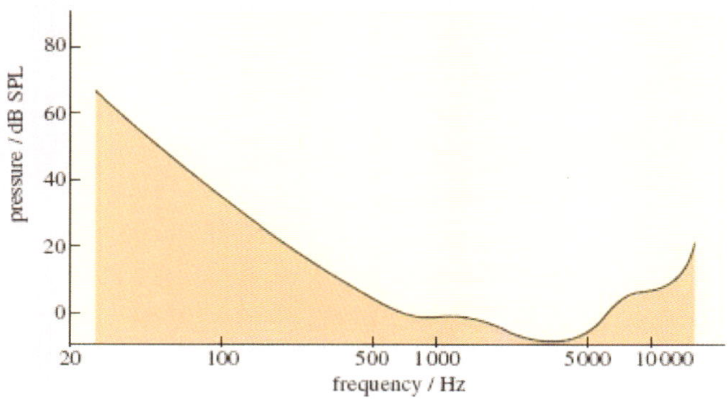

Human auditory thresholds as a function of frequency. Sounds that fall in the shaded region below the curve are below threshold and therefore inaudible

The absolute threshold is the smallest value of some stimulus that a listener can detect. In order to investigate our perceptual capabilities, it is useful to generate an absolute threshold curve, which relates the frequency of a signal to the intensity at which it can be detected by the ear. is a plot of the thresholds of hearing for a range of frequencies.

This means that people are therefore most sensitive to tones of frequencies around 3000 Hz, with sensitivities decreasing for tones that are either higher or lower in frequency. There will be very high and very low frequencies to which, no matter how intense the sinusoidal wave, the auditory system is insensitive. These frequency limits define the bounds of the auditory system's sensitivity to frequency.

In order to generate an audibility curve like that shown in, you would determine the level required for a listener to detect the presence of a sinusoidal wave at each of many frequencies. One method of doing this involves delivering the sound using loudspeakers and measuring the sound pressure at the entrance to the auditory meatus at threshold. A threshold measured in this way is known as a minimum audible field (MAF). In contrast when sounds are delivered through earphones the threshold measured is called the minimum audible pressure (MAP). MAP thresholds are plotted as a function of frequency in.

The threshold sound levels displayed in produce extremely small physical displacements at both the tympanic and basilar membranes. In humans, the sound level of frequencies to which we are most sensitive cause movements of the basilar membrane of about 0.2 nm – about the diameter of two hydrogen atoms.

Shows auditory thresholds for young people. As we grow older, we become less sensitive to stimuli of all frequencies, but the maximum hearing losses occur for high frequency tones.

Factors That Can Influence the Absolute Threshold

While the absolute threshold is often thought of purely in terms of sensation and perception, a number of factors can play a role including expectations, motivations, and thoughts. For example, if you are expecting to hear a noise, you might be more likely to detect it at lower levels than you would if you do not expect to hear the noise.

Researchers have found that women tend to have lower absolute threshold than men, meaning they are better able to detect lower levels of sight, smell, taste, touch, and sound. Introverted people have also been found to be better able to detect stimulus levels at lower levels. However, absolute thresholds are also prone to change as people grow older. When people are younger, they are able to detect energy levels at lower levels but require greater stimulation to detect these same stimuli when they are older.

References

- Daniel Schacter; Daniel Gilbert; Daniel Wegner (2011). "Sensation and Perception". In Charles Linsmeiser. Psychology. Worth Publishers. pp. 158–159. ISBN 978-1-4292-3719-2

- Jeffress L.A. (1948). "A place theory of sound localization". Journal of Comparative and Physiological Psychology. 41: 35–39. doi:10.1037/h0061495. PMID 18904764
- What-is-hearing: hearingaidknow.com, Retrieved 29 June 2018
- Hauser, Marc D. (1998). The evolution of communication. MIT Press. p. 190. ISBN 978-0-262-58155-4. Retrieved 24 May 2011
- Shupak A. Sharoni Z. Yanir Y. Keynan Y. Alfie Y. Halpern P. (January 2005). "Underwater Hearing and Sound Localization with and without an Air Interface". Otology & Neurotology. 26 (1): 127–130. doi:10.1097/00129492-200501000-00023
- Human-hearing-range-what-can-you-hear: global.widex.com, Retrieved 19 April 2018
- William Yost (2003). "Audition". In Alice F. Healy; Robert W. Proctor. Handbook of Psychology: Experimental psychology. John Wiley and Sons. p. 130. ISBN 978-0-471-39262-0
- Rayleigh L. XII. On our perception of sound direction[J]. The London, Edinburgh, and Dublin Philosophical Magazine and Journal of Science, 1907, 13(74): 214-232
- Sound-localization, medicine-and-dentistry: sciencedirect.com, Retrieved 29 June 2018
- Deutsch, Diana (1999). The psychology of music. Gulf Professional Publishing. p. 153. ISBN 978-0-12-213565-1. Retrieved 24 May 2011
- Musicant A D, Butler R A. The influence of pinnae-based spectral cues on sound localization[J]. The Journal of the Acoustical Society of America, 1984, 75(4): 1195-1200
- What-is-the-absolute-threshold-279522: verywellmind.com, Retrieved 24 May 2018
- Beyer, Robert T. (1999). Sounds of our times : two hundred years of acoustics. New York: Springer. ISBN 978-0-387-98435-3

2

Auditory System

The sensory organs and the auditory parts of the sensory system, whose proper functioning is essential for the sense of hearing or the perception of sound, comprise the auditory system. This chapter has been carefully written to provide an easy understanding of the structure of the auditory system with an emphasis on the outer, middle and inner ear as well as the neuronal structure and the mechanism of the neuronal encoding of sound.

The auditory system is one of the engineering masterpieces of the human body. At the heart of the system is an array of miniature acoustical detectors packed into a space no larger than a pea. These detectors can faithfully transduce vibrations as small as the diameter of an atom, and they can respond a thousand times faster than visual photoreceptors. Such rapid auditory responses to acoustical cues facilitate the initial orientation of the head and body to novel stimuli, especially those that are not initially within the field of view. Although humans are highly visual creatures, much human communication is mediated by the auditory system; indeed, loss of hearing can be more socially debilitating than blindness. From a cultural perspective, the auditory system is essential not only to language, but also to music, one of the most aesthetically sophisticated forms of human expression. For these and other reasons, audition represents a fascinating and especially important aspect of sensation, and more generally of brain function.

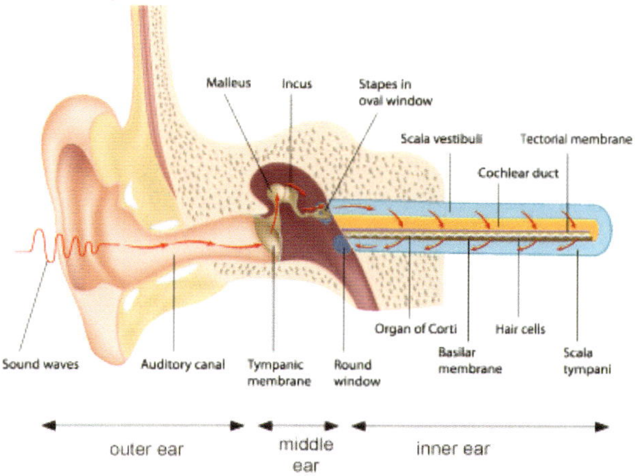

Figure: anatomy of human ear.

The human auditory system is a real wonder - with two compact auditive sensor organs - the ears - at either side of the head, connected with a string of high speed nerve fibers to the brain stem. The brain stem is the central connecting point of the brain connecting the human body's nervous system inputs (such as audio, vision) and outputs (such as muscle control) to the other areas of the brain. The brain stem redirects the audio information from the ears to a section of the brain that is specialised in audio processing: the auditory cortex.

The Auditory System

Although everything in our ear is connected, our auditory systems are divided into three parts: the outer ear, middle ear and inner ear. Each part serves a different function and is essential to our ability to hear properly.

Outer Ear

When we think of hearing, we usually imagine the outer ear – the part you can see. It includes:

- The pinna, or cartilage auricle that extends outside our head;
- The ear canal;
- The tympanic membrane (the outer layer of the eardrum).

Function of Outer Ear

The pinna's shape is designed to collect sound waves and pass them through the ear canal to the tympanic membrane, where sound then enters the middle ear.

Middle Ear

The middle ear is separated from the outer ear by the eardrum. This chamber of the ear is full of air and includes the following structures:

- The ear drum;
- The ossicles, which are three different bones;
    - The malleus (shaped like a hammer, this bone connects to the eardrum);
    - The incus (shaped like an anvil, this bone unites the incus and stapes);
    - The stapes (shaped like a stirrup, this bone transfers the sound to the cochlea).

Function of Middle Ear

Once the sound hits the eardrum, it begins to vibrate. Because all these systems are connected, this in turn causes the ossicles to move. They turn sound waves into a mechanical vibration. The last bone, the stapes, transfers these vibrations to the inner ear.

Inner Ear

This is the final part of the auditory system where sound is changed to an electrical signal the brain can read and interpret. The systems here include:

- The semicircular canals for balance and proprioception.
- The cochlea (a spiral structure made of fluid filled tubes separated by thin membranes. One of the most important parts of the cochlea is the basilar membrane and the organ of Corti which covers it).
- The eighth cranial or vestibulocochlear nerve.

Function of Inner Ear

The inner ear serves two functions – balance and hearing.

Outer Ear

The outer ear comes in all types of shapes and sizes. This structure helps to give each of us our unique appearance.

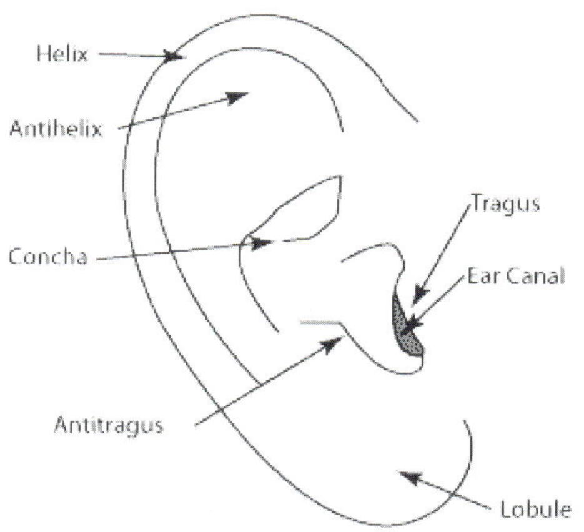

The outer ear is made up of cartilage and skin. There are three different parts to the outer ear; the tragus, helix and the lobule.

The outer ear is the external part of the ear, which collects sound waves and directs them into the ear.

Pinna

What is the pinna? The pinna is the only visible part of the ear (the auricle) with its special helical shape. It is the first part of the ear that reacts with sound. The function of the pinna is to act as a kind of funnel which assists in directing the sound further into the ear. Without this funnel the sound waves would take a more direct route into the auditory canal. This would be both difficult and wasteful as much of the sound would be lost making it harder to hear and understand the sounds.

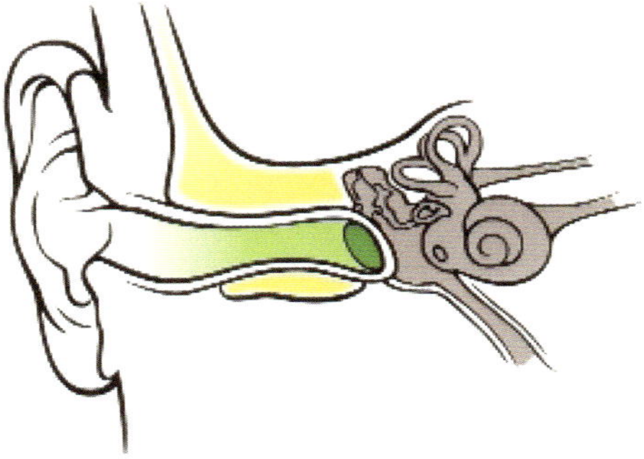

The pinna is essential due to the difference in pressure inside and outside the ear. The resistance of the air is higher inside the ear than outside because the air inside the ear is compressed and thus under greater pressure.

In order for the sound waves to enter the ear in the best possible way the resistance must not be too high. This is where the pinna helps by overcoming the difference in pressure inside and outside the ear. The pinna functions as a kind of intermediate link which makes the transition smoother and less brutal allowing more sound to pass into the auditory canal (meatus).

Ear Canal

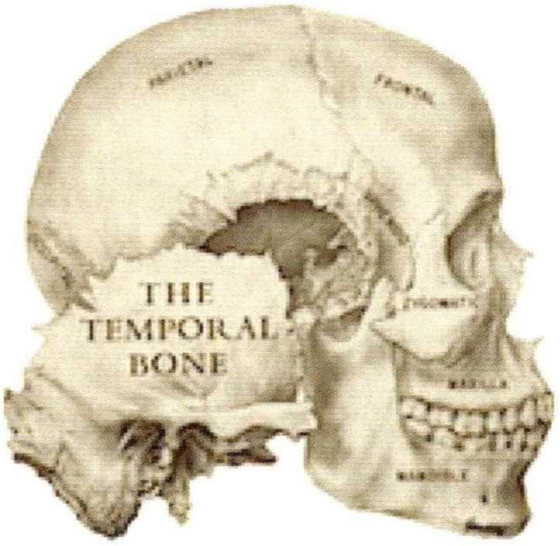

Bones of the skull. The ear canal is housed in the temporal bone.

The ear canal is housed in the temporal bone.

Ear Canal Anatomy

The outer ear (Figure) consists of the auricle (pinna) and the external auditory meatus (ear canal). It ends at the tympanic membrane (ear drum). The ear canal itself is shorter than this, and is essentially a skin-lined cul-de-sac that extends from the aperture (opening) of the ear canal to the tympanic membrane (eardrum).

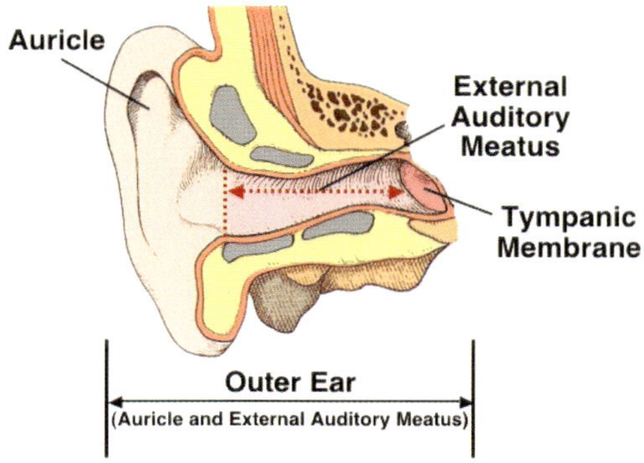

Outer ear, consisting of the auricle and the external auditory meatus (canal). The external auditory meatus extends from the aperture (opening) of the ear canal to the tympanic membrane (shown by the dotted line).

Ear Canal Physiology

The primary function of the ear canal is to serve as a conduit for the passage of sounds to the tympanic membrane (TM). It serves also to protect the middle and inner ears from external trauma by impeding (using distance, shape, and chemical composition) the entry of foreign objects, and by mediating fluctuations in environmental temperatures.

Ear Canal Skeletal Structure

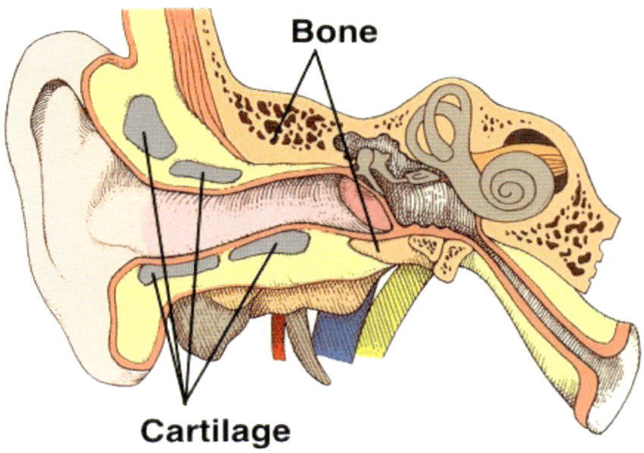

Figure: The skeletal structure of the external auditory meatus consists of cartilage distally, and bone medially.

The skeletal structure of the ear canal (external auditory meatus) consists of elastic cartilage laterally (cartilaginous portion) and bone medially (osseous, or bony portion). This is essentially the same for all individuals, although considerable variation in size, shape, and orientation occurs.

The narrowest part of the ear canal (isthmus) is located near the junction of the cartilaginous and bony canals. The cartilage of the ear canal is continuous with that of the auricle (pinna). Medially, the cartilage is firmly attached to the bony canal. Figure provides measurements of the range of vertical and horizontal dimensions of the isthmus.

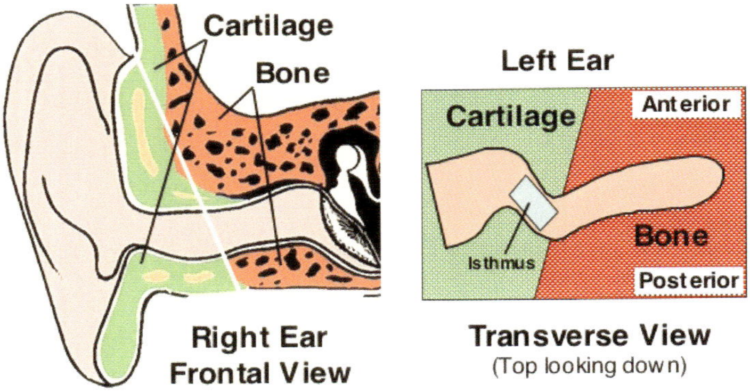

Cartilaginous versus osseous (bony) sections of the external auditory meatus

The cartilaginous part of the ear canal constitutes approximately the outer one-third (mostly) to almost one-half of the total length, but this varies among individuals.

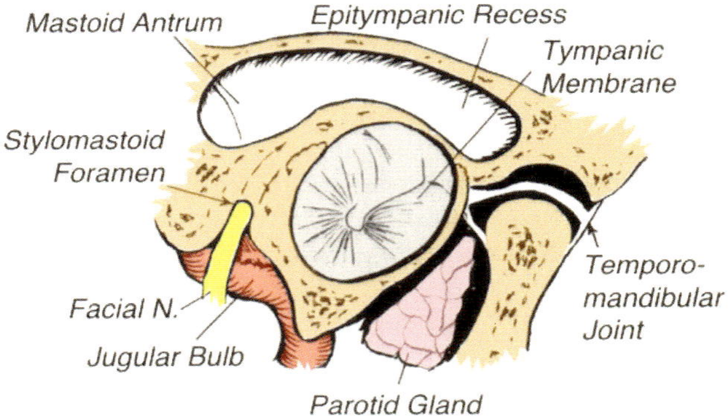

Adjoining structures/areas to the external auditory meatus (right ear), as viewed from the aperture of the ear canal toward the tympanic membrane.

The medial one-third to one-half of the ear canal is osseous (bone) and is oriented in a forward and downward direction. The downward (and inward) orientation is displayed in on the left image, and identified by the white line. The right image of shows that the posterior (and superior, as shown in the left image) portion of the ear canal has greater osseous lining. The ear canal is slightly concave posteriorly so that the ear canal as a whole is slightly S-shaped when viewed from the top. However, there is considerable variation in the configuration and size. Posterosuperiorly, the bony meatus is related from within out to structures of the mastoid bone. Inferiorly, the meatus is in close relation to the jugular bulb, as well as close (posteroinferior) to the facial nerve.

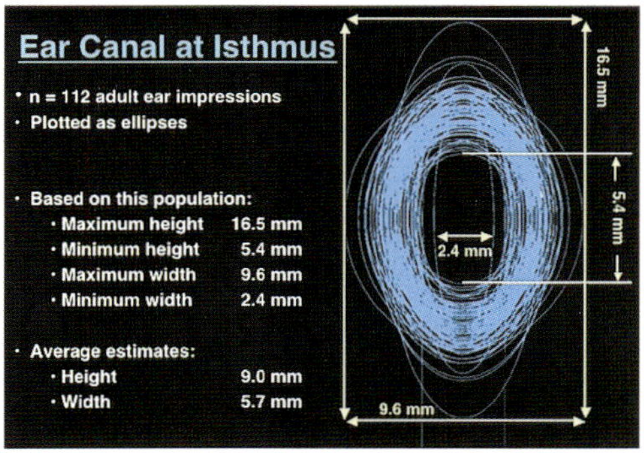

Range of vertical and horizontal measurements of the isthmus taken from 112 impressions made on live subjects.

The middle third of the ear canal is graduated between bone and cartilage, with bone having greater impact along the posterior wall of the canal. The bony meatus is related anteriorly and inferiorly to the parotid (salivary) gland and to the temporomandibular joint . Condyloid movements of the ramus of the mandible,

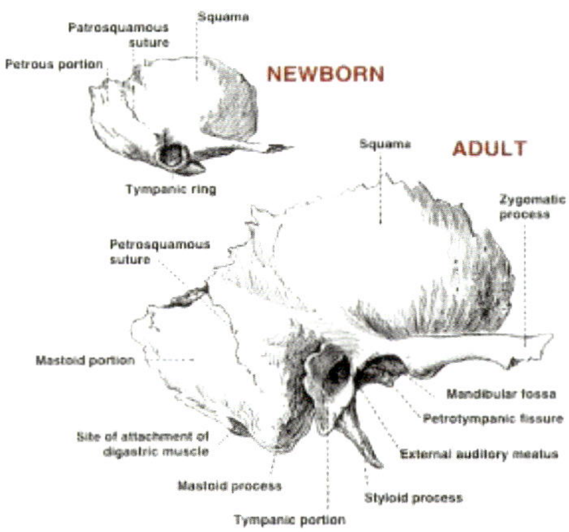

Temporal bones of newborn and adult, showing differences, with special emphasis on the bony walls of the ear canal opening. In the newborn, the tympanic ring is short and incomplete.

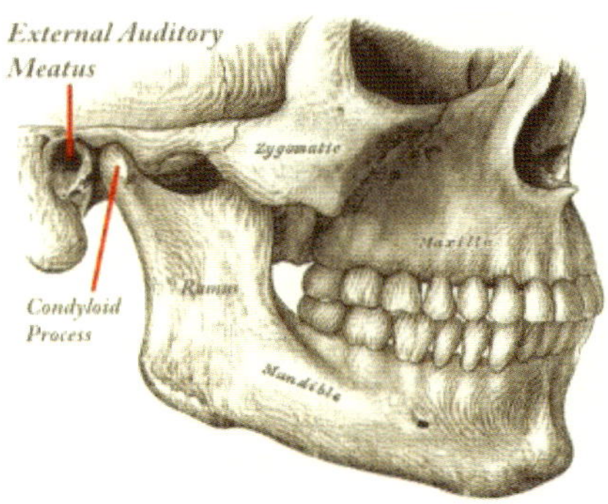

The condyloid process of the ramus of the mandible articulates just anterior to the external auditory meatus, resulting in dimensional changes in the ear canal during jaw movement, regardless of the purpose (speaking, mastication, etc).

as in speech or mastication, can be transmitted to the cartilaginous portion because of the proximity of the mandible to the ear canal.

Eardrum

As the sound makes its way inside of the ear canal, it ends up vibrating the tympanic membrane, which is also known as the eardrum. Your eardrum is essentially a very fine piece of skin, which is less than a half of an inch wide. It is located in between the middle ear and the ear canal.

The Eustachian tube connects the middle ear into the throat. Due to the amount of air from within the atmosphere, your outer ear and the air pressure upon both of your eardrums will remain consistent. It is because of this balance that your eardrums are able to move back and forth with ease.

The eardrums are extremely sensitive and rigid. Even the smallest of fluctuations in air pressure will cause it to move back and forth. It is connected to the tensor tympani muscle, which is constantly working to pull it inside. This action helps to keep the whole membrane tight so that it will vibrate, regardless of what direction the sound wave is coming from.

This miniscule piece of skin acts identical to that of the diaphragm within a microphone. The drum is pushed back and forth because of the rarefactions and the compressions of the different sound waves. Louder sounds cause the eardrum to move at an increased distance, while the higher pitched sounds cause it to move at an increased rate of speed.

Your eardrum also works to protect your inner ear from being exposed to any loud and low pitched sounds. Whenever the brain receives any signals for noises, the eardrum will have some form of a reflex. The stapedius and tensor tympani muscles will end up contracting all of a sudden.

Due to the contractions, the eardrum will end up pulling the bones within the ear in opposite directions, which causes the eardrum to become more rigid in nature. Whenever this occurs, the ear will not receive the level of noise needed at the lower end of the speech spectrum, which causes the loud noises to be lowered in sound.

Beyond just protecting your ear, this reflex ends up helping you to concentrate on your hearing. It helps to mask out the loud noises in the background to allow you to focus your attention on the higher pitched sounds. Amongst other factors, this also helps you to carry on a conversation whenever you are in an extremely noisy environment, such as a rock concert or an auditorium.

The reflex also jumps into motion to help you hear when you begin talking. Otherwise, you would only end up hearing the sound of your own voice and it would cancel out anyone else who may be talking around you.

The eardrum is essentially the main element for sensing sounds in your entire ear. All of the other components of your ear only work to pass the information along that have already been compiled at the eardrum. As complex as the hearing process is, this is only a portion of it and there is a lot more that goes into allowing us to hear the sounds in the environment on a regular basis.

Middle Ear

Parts of the Middle Ear

The middle ear can be split into two; the tympanic cavity and epitympanic recess.

The tympanic cavity lies medially to the tympanic membrane. It contains the majority of the bones of the middle ear. The epitympanic recess is found superiorly, near the mastoid air cells.

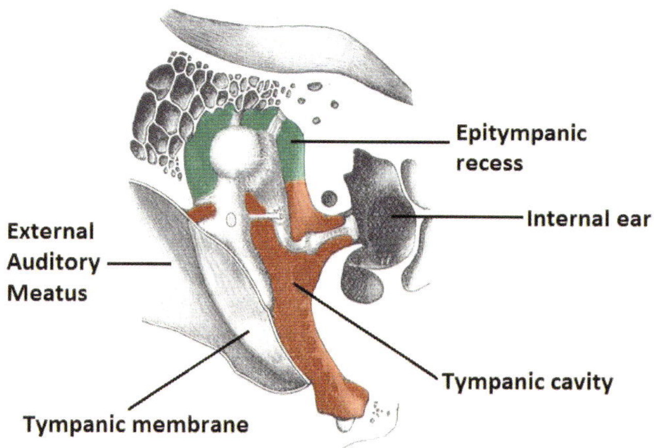

The middle ear. The two main parts of the middle ear have been labelled.

Borders

The middle ear can be visualised as a rectangular box, with a roof and floor, medial and lateral walls and anterior and posterior walls.

- Roof – Formed by a thin bone from the petrous part of the temporal bone. It separates the middle ear from the middle cranial fossa.
- Floor – Known as the jugular wall, it consists of a thin layer of bone, which separates the middle ear from the internal jugular vein
- Lateral Wall – This is made up of the tympanic membrane and the lateral wall of the epitympanic recess.

- Medial Wall – Formed by the lateral wall of the internal ear. It contains a prominent bulge, produced by the facial nerve as it travels nearby.
- Anterior Wall – The anterior wall is a thin bony plate with two openings; for the auditory tube and the tensor tympani muscle. It separates the middle ear from the internal carotid artery.
- Posterior Wall – Also known as the mastoid wall, it consists of a bony partition between the tympanic cavity and the mastoid air cells. Superiorly, there is a hole in this partition, allowing the two areas to communication. This hole is known as the aditus to the mastoid antrum.

Bones

The bones of the middle ear are called the auditory ossicles. They are the malleus, incus and stapes. They are connected in a chain-like manner, linking the tympanic membrane to the oval window of the internal ear.

The malleus is the largest and most lateral of the ear bones, attaching to the tympanic membrane, via the handle of malleus. The head of the malleus lies in the epitympanic recess, where it articulates with the next auditory ossicle, the incus.

The next bone, the incus, consists of a body and two limbs. The body articulates with the malleus, the short limb attaches to the posterior wall of the middle, and the long limb joins the last of the ossicles; the stapes.

The stapes is the smallest bone in the human body. It joins the incus to the oval window of the inner ear. It is stirrup-shaped, with a head, two limbs, and a base. The head articulates with the incus, and the base joins the oval window.

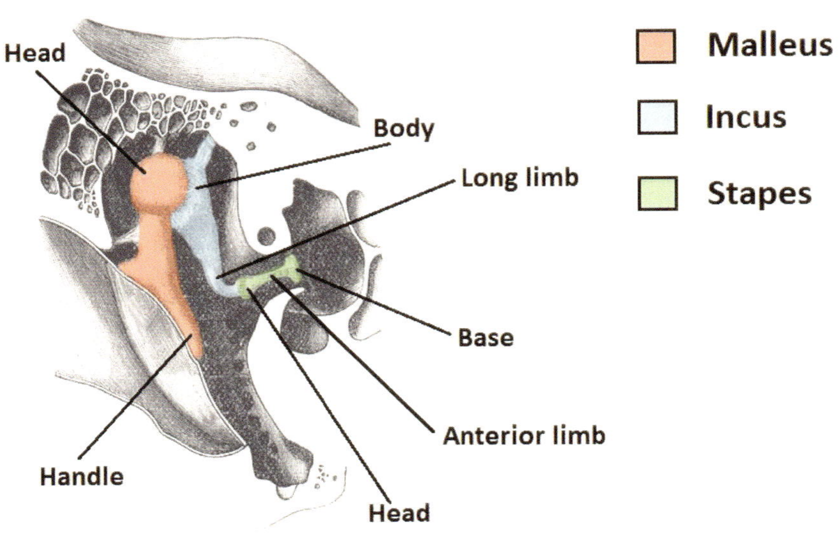

Bones of the middle ear.

Mastoid Air Cells

The mastoid air cells are located posterior to epitympanic recess. They are a collection of air-filled spaces in the mastoid process of the temporal bone. The air cells are contained within a cavity called the mastoid antrum. The mastoid antrum communicates with the middle ear via the aditus to mastoid antrum.

The mastoid air cells act as a 'buffer system' of air – releasing air into the tympanic cavity when the pressure is too low.

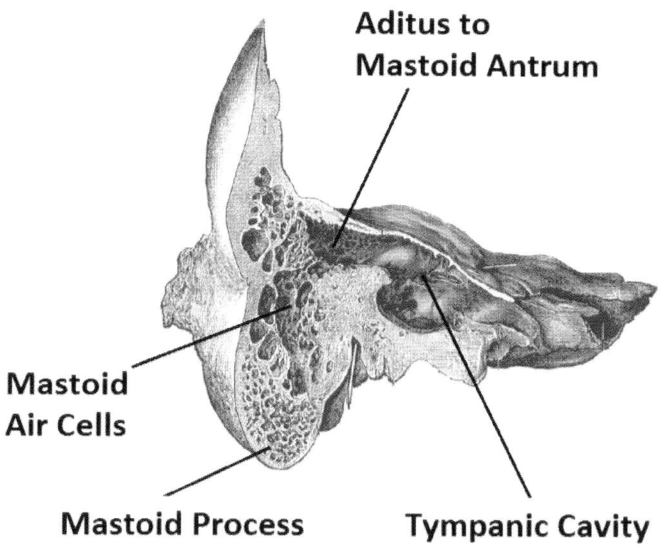

Coronal section of temporal bone, showing the mastoid air cells in more detail

Muscles

There are two muscles which serve a protective function in the middle ear; the tensor tympani and stapedius. They contract in response to loud noise, inhibiting the vibrations of the malleus, incus and stapes, and reducing the transmission of sound to the inner ear. This action is known as the acoustic reflex.

The tensor tympani originates from the auditory tube and attaches to the handle of malleus, pulling it medially when contracting. It is innervated by a branch of the mandibular nerve. The stapedius muscle attaches to the stapes, and is innervated by the facial nerve.

Auditory Tube

The auditory tube (eustachian tube) is a cartilaginous and bony tube that connects the middle ear to the nasopharynx. It acts to equalise the pressure of the middle ear to that of the external auditory meatus.

It extends from the anterior wall of the middle ear, in anterior, medioinferior direction, opening onto the lateral wall of the nasopharynx. In joining the two structures, it is a pathway by which an upper respiratory infection can spread into the middle ear.

Acoustic Reflex

The acoustic reflex, also known as the stapedius reflex refers to an involuntary muscle contraction of the stapedius muscle in response to a high-intensity sound stimulus. Due to ease of administration and information yielded, the acoustic reflex is considered one of the most powerful differential diagnostic audiological procedures.

Acoustic reflexes do not measure hearing threshold. Rather, they measure reflected energy which is a function of stapedius muscle contraction; it allows one to indirectly assess the middle ear, cochlea and neural innervation of the stapedius muscle.

As the acoustic reflex is involuntary and bilateral, it is replicable and provides valuable diagnostic information when comparing the amount of reflected energy according to signal intensity, as well as the presence of ipsilateral and bilateral acoustic reflexes.

Premise Behind Instrumentation

An acoustic stimulus is presented to the external auditory canal; energy is transferred from the ear canal through the middle ear, some of which is reflected and some absorbed by the tympanic membrane and external ear structures.

The premise behind the immittance instrumentation used to measure the acoustic reflex is the ability to accurately measure changes in reflected energy occurring from stiffening of the tympanic membrane as a result of contraction of the stapedius muscle (For the premise behind tympanometry). The amount of reflected and absorbed energy varies depending on the admittance/impedance (flow/resistance) of energy within the system and the complex interaction between the ear structures.

The presence of reflexes within normal intensity limits is consistent with normal middle ear and brainstem function and suggests that auditory sensitivity is not significantly impaired. An elevated or absent acoustic reflex threshold is consistent with a middle ear disorder, hearing loss in the stimulated ear, and/or interruption of neural innervation of the stapedius muscle.

Anatomy and Physiology

Neural mechanisms mediate the acoustic reflex that results in involuntary stapedius muscle contraction stiffening the stapes within the middle ear. It is presumed that the physiologic reason for the reflex is that it serves as an inhibitory response to reduce the sound intensities reaching the inner ear by as much as 20 dB evoked when individuals vocalise (Møller, 2000).

As is illustrated in Figure, once a high intensity auditory stimulus is initiated and reaches the cochleae, neural impulses from the auditory nerves (CN VIII) ascend from both cochleae to each ipsilateral ventral cochlear nucleus (VCN). From VCN the reflex has two main neural pathways: one passes from the VCN directly to the ipsilateral facial motor nucleus (CN VII) that directly innervates the stapedius muscle via the facial nerve and its stapedius branch; the other passes from the VCN to the superior olivary complex (SOC) before the impulses cross at the brainstem to innervate both ipsilateral and contralateral facial motor nuclei.

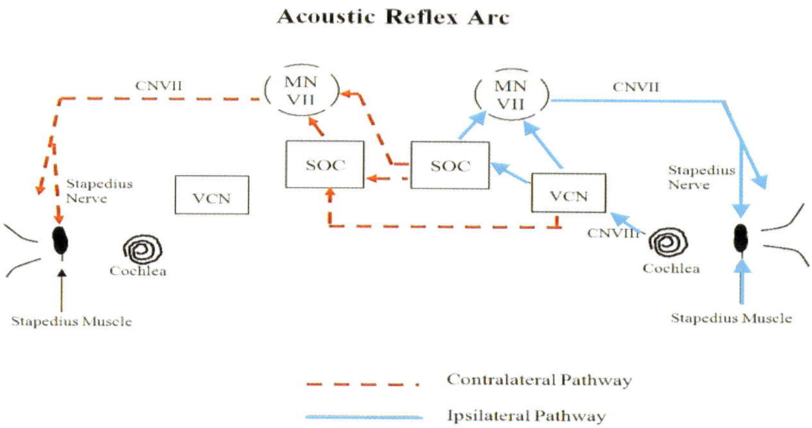

Schematic of the acoustic reflex neural pathways. CNVII; CNVIII; MNVII; SOC; VCN. Dashed lines represent the contralateral pathway and solid lines represent ipsilateral pathway of acoustic reflex

Contraction of the stapedius muscle stiffens the middle ear ossicles and tilts the stapes in the oval window of the cochlea; this effectively decreases the vibrational energy transmitted to the cochlea. Stapedius muscle contraction is clinically apparent by a marked change in the impedance properties of the middle ear.

It is important to realize that a bilateral acoustic reflex occurs i.e. stimulating one ear (ipsilateral ear) elicits an acoustic reflex in both the ipsilateral and contralateral ears.

Acoustic Threshold

An acoustic reflex threshold is the lowest intensity level at which an acoustic reflex is elicited at each frequency for each ear.

Stapedius muscle contraction increases as the stimulus intensity is increased; it is therefore possible to determine acoustic reflex thresholds by incrementally increasing the stimulus by 5 dB steps, beginning at 80 dB HL, until a contraction occurs . With a normally functioning middle ear and cochlea, an acoustic reflex is elicited contralaterally at four frequencies (500, 1000, 2000, 4000 Hz), and ipsilaterally at two frequencies (1000, 2000 Hz) when stimulus intensities of 85-90 dB HL (hearing level) are delivered to the ear canal.

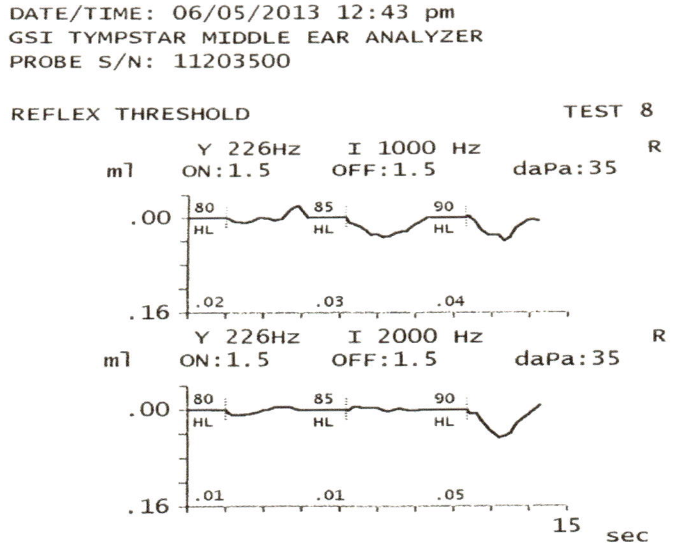

Example (right ear) of acoustic reflex threshold obtained from an immittance instrument. Results shown would indicate 85 & 90 dB HL thresholds for 1000 and 2000 Hz respectively, which would be expected for a normal ear

In a normal ear, after an initial contraction the strength increases with each sequential increase of signal intensity until a plateau is reached. Threshold is defined as the lowest acoustic stimulus intensity elicited with a deflection magnitude of at least 0.03ml. As seen in the magnitude of deflections in Figure, thresholds for both frequencies assessed clearly fall within the criteria of at least 0.03ml deflection. To identify a threshold it is advisable to confirm the magnitude of the deflection with a repeat presentation. Once a threshold has been established at one frequency, the intensity is recorded, and the other frequencies are then assessed. During quick screening it is not unusual to assess an acoustic reflex threshold at only one frequency and a single set intensity (~95 or 100 dB HL. An ipsilateral acoustic reflex threshold tends to be attained at a slightly lower intensity stimulus than an acoustic reflex threshold elicited by a contralateral stimulus.

Factors Affecting Acoustic Reflexes

- Ipsilateral conductive hearing loss: Anything that obstructs transmission of a sound signal to the cochlea in the stimulated ear results in reduced or absent contraction of the stapedius muscles. Middle ear disorders therefore easily mask an acoustic reflex. Forty percent of patients with conductive hearing loss of >20 dB HL do not have an acoustic reflex. Once conductive hearing loss reaches 40 dB HL, about 80% of patients do not have a reflex (Jerger, Anthony, Jerger and Mauldin, 1974).
- Ipsilateral sensorineural hearing loss: This may obstruct transmission of a

signal beyond the cochlea of the stimulated ear and usually causes reduced or absent contraction of the stapedius muscles. However, because of recruitment of loudness in cochlear sensorineural hearing loss, acoustic reflexes may occur even within the expected normal or partially elevated intensity range in the presence of mild or moderate-to-severe sensorineural hearing loss.

- Stapes fixation: The stapes footplate is more-or-less fixed to the surrounding bone with otosclerosis (and sometimes with tympanosclerosis). This may interfere with the acoustic reflex in two ways: it causes a conductive hearing loss; and reduced mobility of the stapes prevents stiffening of the tympanic membrane when the stapedius muscle contracts .
- Ossicular disarticulation: As with otosclerosis, it causes a conductive hearing loss, and if located lateral to the stapes, prevents stiffening of the ossicles and tympanic membrane when the stapedius muscle contracts.
- Middle ear effusion: This causes a conductive hearing loss, and reduces compliance of the tympanic membrane and middle ear structures and may mask the presence of an acoustic reflex.
- Tympanic membrane perforation: This causes a conductive hearing loss. Furthermore, due to the perforation, changes in compliance caused by contraction of the stapedius muscle cannot be measured.
- Negative/abnormal middle ear pressure: To maximize the likelihood that a reflex will be detected, the pressure on either side of the tympanic membrane has to be equal for the tympanic membrane to be at or near the point of maximum compliance for further explanation). This necessitates one to match the peak pressure of the tympanogram to the actual middle ear pressure so that valid acoustic reflex threshold values may be obtained.
- Facial nerve dysfunction: The stapedius muscle is innervated by the facial nerve. Contraction of the stapedius muscle has to occur for both ipsi- and contralateral acoustic reflexes.

Interpretation of Acoustic Reflexes

Acoustic reflexes may be reported as:

- Ipsilateral: Reflex recorded in ear to which auditory stimulus is presented;
- Contralateral: Reflex recorded in ear contralateral to which auditory stimulus is presented;
- Partially present: Reflex present at some frequencies and absent at others;

- Elevated threshold: Reflex thresholds elicited >100 dB HL;
- Absent reflex: No reflex elicited.

Partial or elevated reflex thresholds may indicate the presence of hearing loss at the frequencies where they are specifically absent.

Absent reflexes have also been observed in individuals with normal or near-normal hearing, which may then indicate middle ear disease or neurological involvement of the 8th cranial nerve, such as in pontine angle tumours and auditory neuropathy, or neurological involvement of the 7th cranial nerve. With facial nerve paralysis, the absence of acoustic reflexes in the presence of normal middle ear function suggests a lesion in the neural pathway proximal to the stapedius nerve, whereas the presence of an acoustic reflex in patients with facial nerve paralysis suggests that the lesion is distal to the origin of the nerve. A very small percentage of people will have normal auditory sensitivity and absent acoustic reflexes across all frequencies without other identifiable pathology.

Inner Ear

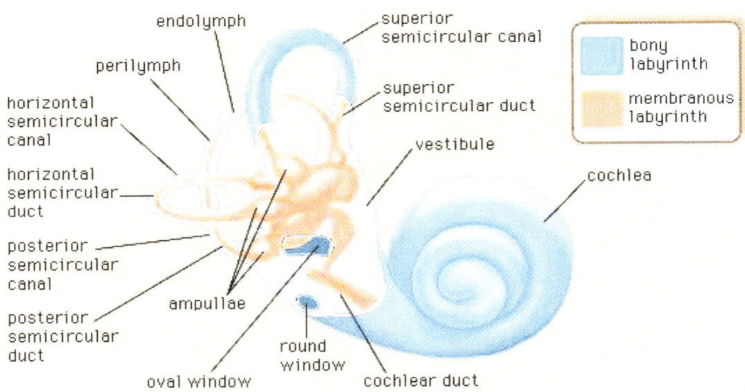

The two labyrinths of the inner ear.
The bony labyrinth is partially cut away to show the membranous labyrinth within.

There are actually two labyrinths of the inner ear, one inside the other, the membranous labyrinth contained within the bony labyrinth. The bony labyrinth consists of a central chamber called the vestibule, the three semicircular canals, and the spirally coiled cochlea. Within each structure, and filling only a fraction of the available space, is a corresponding portion of the membranous labyrinth: the vestibule contains the utricle and saccule, each semicircular canal its semicircular duct, and the cochlea its cochlear duct. Surrounding the membranous labyrinth and filling the remaining space is the watery fluid called perilymph. It is derived from blood plasma and resembles but is not identical with the cerebrospinal fluid of the brain and the aqueous humour of the eye. Like most of the hollow organs, the membranous labyrinth is lined with epithelium (a sheet of specialized cells that covers internal and external body surfaces). It is filled with a fluid called endolymph, which has a markedly different ionic content from perilymph. Because the membranous labyrinth is a closed system, the endolymph and perilymph do not mix.

Vestibule

The two membranous sacs of the vestibule, the utricle and the saccule, are known as the otolith organs. Because they respond to gravitational forces, they are also called gravity receptors. Each sac has on its inner surface a single patch of sensory cells called a macula, which is about 2 mm (0.08 inch) in diameter. The macula monitors the position of the head relative to the vertical. In the utricle the macula projects from the anterior wall of that tubular sac and lies primarily in the horizontal plane. In the saccule the macula is in the vertical plane and directly overlies the bone of the inner wall of the vestibule. In shape it is elongated and resembles the letter J. Each macula consists of neuroepithelium, a layer that is made up of supporting cells and sensory cells, as well as a basement membrane, nerve fibres and nerve endings, and underlying connective tissue. The sensory cells are called hair cells because of the hairlike cilia—stiff nonmotile stereocilia and flexible motile kinocilia—that project from their apical ends. The nerve fibres are from the superior, or vestibular, division of the vestibulocochlear nerve. They pierce the basement membrane and, depending on the type of hair cell, either end on the basal end of the cell or form a calyx, or cuplike structure, that surrounds it.

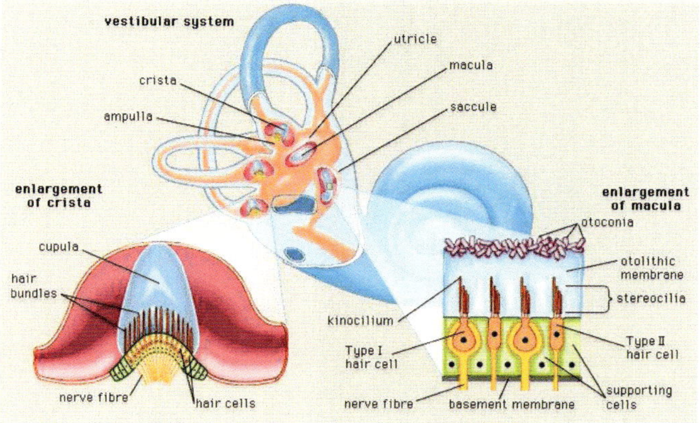

The membranous labyrinth of the vestibular system (centre), which contains the organs of balance, and (lower left) the cristae of the semicircular ducts and (lower right) the maculae of the utricle and saccule.

Each of the hair cells of the vestibular organs is topped by a hair bundle, which consists of about 100 fine nonmotile stereocilia of graded lengths and a single motile kinocilium. The stereocilia are anchored in a dense cuticular plate at the cell's apex. The single kinocilium, which is larger and longer than the stereocilia, rises from a noncuticular area of the cell membrane at one side of the cuticular plate. The longest stereocilia are those closest to the kinocilium; the stereocilia decrease in length in stepwise fashion away from the kinocilium. Minute filamentous strands link the tips and shafts of neighbouring stereocilia to one another. When the hair bundles are deflected—e.g., because of a tilt of the head—the hair cells are stimulated to alter the rate of the nerve impulses that they are constantly sending via the vestibular nerve fibres to the brainstem. Covering the entire macula is a delicate acellular structure, the otolithic, or statolithic, membrane. This membrane is sometimes described as gelatinous, although it has a fibrillar pattern. The surface of the membrane is covered by a blanket of rhombohedral crystals, referred to as otoconia or statoconia, which consist of calcium carbonate in the form of calcite. These crystalline particles, which range in length from 1 to 20 μm (1 μm = 0.000039 inch), are much denser than the membrane—their specific gravity is almost three times that of the membrane and the endolymph—and thus add considerable mass to it.

The vestibular hair cells are of two types: type I cells have a rounded body enclosed by a nerve calyx, and type II cells have a cylindrical body with nerve endings at the base. They form a mosaic on the surface of the maculae, with the type I cells dominating in a curvilinear area (the striola) near the centre of the macula and the cylindrical cells around the periphery. The significance of these patterns is poorly understood, but they may increase sensitivity to slight tiltings of the head.

Semicircular Canals

The three semicircular canals of the bony labyrinth are designated according to their position: superior, horizontal, and posterior. The superior and posterior canals are in diagonal vertical planes that intersect at right angles. Each canal has an expanded end, the ampulla, which opens into the vestibule. The ampullae of the horizontal and superior canals lie close together, just above the oval window, but the ampulla of the posterior canal opens on the opposite side of the vestibule. The other ends of the superior and posterior canals join to form a common stem, or crus, which also opens into the vestibule. Nearby is the mouth of a canal called the vestibular aqueduct, which opens into the cranial cavity. The other end of the horizontal canal has a separate opening into the vestibule. Thus, the vestibule completes the circle for each of the semicircular canals.

Each of the three bony canals and its ampulla enclose a membranous semicircular duct of much smaller diameter that has its own ampulla. The membranous ducts and ampullae follow the same pattern as the canals and ampullae of the bony labyrinth, with their openings into the utricle and with a common crus for the superior and posterior ducts. Like the other parts of the membranous labyrinth, they are filled with endolymph and surrounded by perilymph. The narrow endolymphatic duct passes from the utricle through the vestibular aqueduct into the cranial cavity, carrying excess endolymph to be absorbed by the endolymphatic sac.

Each membranous ampulla contains a saddle-shaped ridge of tissue called the crista, the sensory end organ that extends across it from side to side. The crista is covered by neuroepithelium, with hair cells and supporting cells. From this ridge rises a gelatinous structure, the cupula, which extends to the roof of the ampulla immediately above it, dividing the interior of the ampulla into two approximately equal parts. Like the hair cells of the maculae, the hair cells of the cristae have hair bundles projecting from their apices. The kinocilium and the longest stereocilia extend far up into the substance of the cupula, occupying fine parallel channels. Thus, the cupula is attached at its base to the crista but is free to incline toward or away from the utricle in response to the slightest flow of endolymph or a change in pressure. The tufts of cilia move with the cupula and, depending on the direction of their bending, cause an increase or a decrease in the rate of nerve impulse discharges carried by the vestibular nerve fibres to the brainstem.

Cochlea

Structure of the Cochlea

The cochlea contains the sensory organ of hearing. It bears a striking resemblance to the shell of a snail and in fact takes its name from the Greek word for this object. The cochlea is a spiral tube that is coiled two and one-half turns around a hollow central pillar, the modiolus. It forms a cone approximately 9 mm (0.35 inch) in diameter at its base and 5 mm in height. When stretched out, the spiral tube is approximately 30 mm in length. It is widest—2 mm—at the point where the basal coil opens into the vestibule, and it tapers until it ends blindly at the apex. The otherwise hollow centre of the modiolus contains the cochlear artery and vein, as well as the twisted trunk of fibres of the cochlear nerve. This nerve, a division of the very short vestibulocochlear nerve, enters the base of the modiolus from the brainstem through an opening in the petrous portion of the temporal bone called the internal meatus. The spiral ganglion cells of the cochlear nerve are found in a bony spiral canal winding around the central core.

A thin bony shelf, the osseous spiral lamina, winds around the modiolus like the thread of a screw. It projects about halfway across the cochlear canal, partly dividing it into two compartments, an upper chamber called the scala vestibuli (vestibular ramp) and a lower chamber called the scala tympani (tympanic ramp). The scala vestibuli and scala tympani, which are filled with perilymph, communicate with each other through an opening at the apex of the cochlea, called the helicotrema, which can be seen if the cochlea is sliced longitudinally down the middle. At its basal end, near the middle ear, the scala vestibuli opens into the vestibule. The basal end of the scala tympani ends blindly just below the round window. Nearby is the opening of the narrow cochlear aqueduct, through which passes the perilymphatic duct. This duct connects the interior of the cochlea with the subdural space in the posterior cranial fossa (the rear portion of the floor of the cranial cavity).

A smaller scala, called the cochlear duct (scala media), lies between the larger vestibular and tympanic scalae; it is the cochlear portion of the membranous labyrinth. Filled with endolymph, the cochlear duct ends blindly at both ends—i.e., below the round window and at the apex. In cross section this duct resembles a right triangle. Its base is formed by the osseous spiral lamina and the basilar membrane, which separate the cochlear duct from the scala tympani. Resting on the basilar membrane is the organ of Corti, which contains the hair cells that give rise to nerve signals in response to sound vibrations. The side of the triangle is formed by two tissues that line the bony wall of the cochlea: the stria vascularis, which lines the outer wall of the cochlear duct, and the fibrous spiral ligament, which lies between the stria and the bony wall of the cochlea. A layer of flat cells bounds the stria, separating it from the spiral ligament. The hypotenuse is formed by the transparent vestibular membrane (or Reissner membrane), which consists of only two layers of flattened cells. A low ridge, the spiral limbus, rests on the margin of the osseous spiral lamina. The Reissner membrane stretches from the inner margin of the limbus to the upper border of the stria.

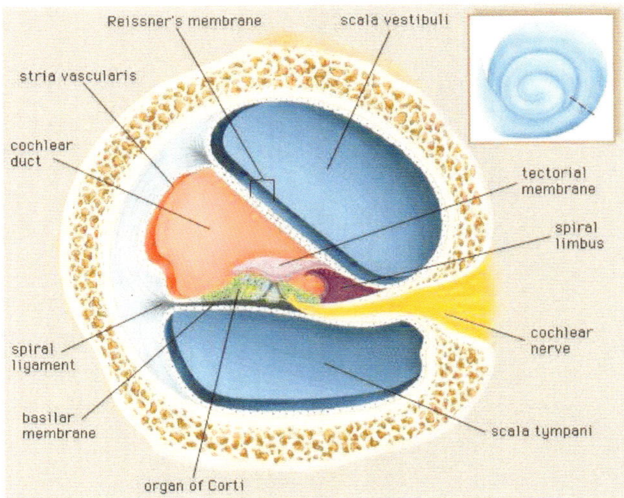

A cross section through one of the turns of the cochlea (inset) showing the scala tympani and scala vestibuli, which contain perilymph, and the cochlear duct, which is filled with endolymph.

The spiral ligament extends above the attachment of the Reissner membrane and is in contact with the perilymph in the scala vestibuli. Extending below the insertion of the basilar membrane, it is in contact with the perilymph of the scala tympani. It contains many stout fibres that anchor the basilar membrane and numerous connective-tissue cells. The structure of the spiral ligament is denser behind the stria than near the upper and lower margins. The spiral ligament, like the adjacent stria, is well supplied with blood vessels. It receives the radiating arterioles that pass outward from the modiolus in bony channels of the roof of the scala vestibuli. Branches from these vessels form a network of capillaries above the junction with the Reissner membrane that may be largely responsible for the formation of the perilymph from the blood plasma. Other branches enter the stria, and still others pass behind it to the spiral prominence. From these separate capillary networks, which are not interconnected, small veins descending below the attachment of the basilar membrane collect blood and deliver it to the spiral vein in the floor of the scala tympani.

At the lower margin of the stria is the spiral prominence, a low ridge parallel to the basilar membrane that contains its own set of longitudinally directed capillary vessels. Below the prominence is the outer sulcus. The floor of the outer sulcus is lined by cells of epithelial origin, some of which send long projections into the substance of the spiral ligament. Between these so-called root cells, capillary vessels descend from the spiral ligament. This region appears to have an absorptive rather than a secretory function, and it may be involved in removing waste materials from the endolymph.

In humans the basilar membrane is about 30 to 35 mm in length. It widens from less than 0.1 mm near its basal end to 0.5 mm near the apex. The basilar membrane is spanned by stiff elastic fibres that are connected at their basal ends in the modiolus. Their distal ends are embedded in the membrane but are not actually attached, which allows them to vibrate. The fibres decrease in calibre and increase in length from the basal end of the cochlea near the middle ear to the apex, so that the basilar membrane as a whole decreases remarkably in stiffness from base to apex. Furthermore, at the basal end the osseous spiral lamina is broader, the stria vascularis wider, and the spiral ligament stouter than at the apex. In contrast, however, the mass of the organ of Corti is least at the base and greatest at the apex. Thus, a certain degree of tuning is provided in the structure of the cochlear duct and its contents. With greater stiffness and less mass, the basal end is more attuned to the sounds of higher frequencies. Decreased stiffness and increased mass render the apical end more responsive to lower frequencies.

Beneath the fibrillar layer of the basilar membrane is the acellular ground substance of the membrane. This layer is covered in turn by a single layer of spindle-shaped mesothelial cells, which have long processes arranged longitudinally and parallel, facing the scala tympani and forming the tympanic lamella that is in contact with the perilymph.

Capillary blood vessels are found on the underside of the tympanic lip of the limbus and, in some species, including the guinea pig and humans, within the basilar membrane, beneath the tunnel. These vessels, called spiral vessels, do not enter the organ of Corti but are thought to supply most of the oxygen and other nutrients to its cells. Although the outer spiral vessel is seldom found in adult animals of certain species such as the dog, cat, and rat and is not found in the basilar membrane of every adult human, it is present in the human fetus. Its impressive diameter in the fetus suggests that it is an important channel for blood delivery to the developing organ of Corti.

Endolymph and Perilymph

The perilymph, which fills the space within the bony labyrinth surrounding the membranous labyrinth, is similar, but not identical, in composition to other extracellular fluids of the body, such as cerebrospinal fluid. The concentration of sodium ions in the perilymph is high (about 150 milliequivalents per litre), and that of potassium ions is low (about 5 milliequivalents per litre), as is true of other extracellular fluids. Like these fluids, the perilymph is apparently formed locally from the blood plasma by transport mechanisms that selectively allow substances to cross the walls of the capillaries. Although it is anatomically possible for cerebrospinal fluid to enter the cochlea by way of the perilymphatic duct, experimental studies have made it appear unlikely that the cerebrospinal fluid is involved in the normal production of perilymph.

The membranous labyrinth is filled with endolymph, which is unique among extracellular fluids of the body, including the perilymph, in that its potassium ion concentration is higher (about 140 milliequivalents per litre) than its sodium ion concentration (about 15 milliequivalents per litre).

The process of formation of the endolymph and the maintenance of the difference in ionic composition between it and perilymph are not yet completely understood. The Reissner membrane forms a selective barrier between the two fluids. Blood-endolymph and blood-perilymph barriers, which control the passage of substances such as drugs from the blood to the inner ear, appear to exist as well. Evidence indicates that the endolymph is produced from perilymph as a result of selective ion transport through the epithelial cells of the Reissner membrane and not directly from the blood. The secretory tissue called the stria vascularis, in the lateral wall of the cochlear duct, is thought to play an important role in maintaining the high ratio of potassium ions to sodium ions in the endolymph. Other tissues of the cochlea, as well as the dark cells of the vestibular organs, which must produce their own endolymph, are also thought to be involved in maintaining the ionic composition of the endolymph. Because the membranous labyrinth is a closed system, the questions of flow and removal of the endolymph are also important. The endolymph is thought to be reabsorbed from the endolymphatic sac, although this appears to be only part of the story. Other cochlear and vestibular tissues may also have important roles in regulating the volume and maintaining the composition of the inner-ear fluids.

Hair Cell

The hair cell is an evolutionary triumph that solves the problem of transforming vibrational energy into an electrical signal. The scale at which the hair cell operates is truly amazing: At the limits of human hearing, hair cells can faithfully detect movements of atomic dimensions and respond in the tens of microseconds. Furthermore, hair cells can adapt rapidly to constant stimuli, thus allowing the listener to extract signals from a noisy background.

The hair cell is a flask-shaped epithelial cell named for the bundle of hairlike processes that protrude from its apical end into the scala media. Each hair bundle contains anywhere from 30 to a few hundred hexagonally arranged stereocilia, with one taller kinocilium . Despite their names, only the kinocilium is a true ciliary structure, with the characteristic two central tubules surrounded by nine doublet tubules . The function of the kinocilium is unclear, and in the cochlea of humans and other mammals it actually disappears shortly after birth . The stereocilia are simpler, containing only an actin cytoskeleton. Each stereocilium tapers where it inserts into the apical membrane, forming a hinge about which each stereocilium pivots . The stereocilia are graded in height and are arranged in a bilaterally symmetric fashion (in vestibular hair cells, this plane runs through the kinocilium). Displacement of the hair bundle parallel to this plane toward the tallest stereocilia depolarizes the hair cell, while movements parallel to this plane toward the shortest stereocilia cause hyperpolarization. In contrast, displacements perpendicular to the plane of symmetry do not alter the hair cell's membrane potential. The hair bundle movements at the threshold of hearing are approximately 0.3 nm, about the diameter of an atom of gold.

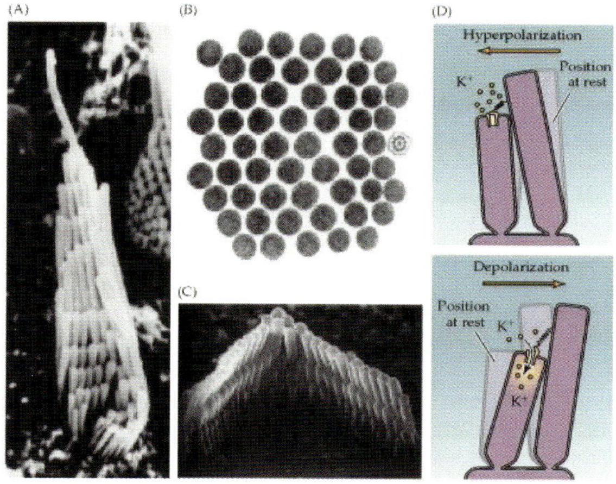

The structure and function of the hair bundle. The vestibular hair bundles shown here resemble those of cochlear hair cells, except for the presence of the kinocilium, which disappears in the mammalian cochlea shortly after birth:

(A) The hair bundle of a guinea pig vestibular hair cell. This view shows the increasing height leading to the kinocilium (arrow).

(B) Cross section through the vestibular hair bundle shows the 9 + 2 array of microtubules in the kinocilium (on right), which contrasts with the simpler actin filament structure of the stereocilia.

(C) Scanning electron micrograph of a guinea pig cochlear outer hair cell bundle viewed along the plane of mirror symmetry. Note the graded lengths of the stereocilia, and the absence of a kinocilium.

(D) Diagram of the stereocilia and tip links, which, when stretched by movement toward the kinocilium, open channels that generate a depolarizing current. When compressed, these same structures lead to hyperpolarization of the hair cell.

Hair cells can convert the displacement of the stereociliary bundle into an electrical potential in as little as 10 microseconds; indeed, such speed is required to faithfully transduce high-frequency signals and enable the accurate localization of the source of the sound. The need for microsecond resolution places certain constraints on the transduction mechanism, ruling out the relatively slow second messenger pathways used in visual and olfactory transduction; a direct, mechanically gated transduction channel is needed to operate this quickly. Evidently the filamentous structures that connect the tips of adjacent stereocilia, known as tip links, directly open cation-selective transduction channels when stretched, allowing K^+ ions to flow into the cell. As the linked stereocilia pivot from side to side, the tension on the tip link varies, modulating the ionic flow and resulting in a graded receptor potential that follows the movements of the stereocilia. The tip link model also explains why only deflections along the axis of the hair bundle activate transduction channels, since tip links join adjacent stereocilia along the axis directed toward the tallest stereocilia .

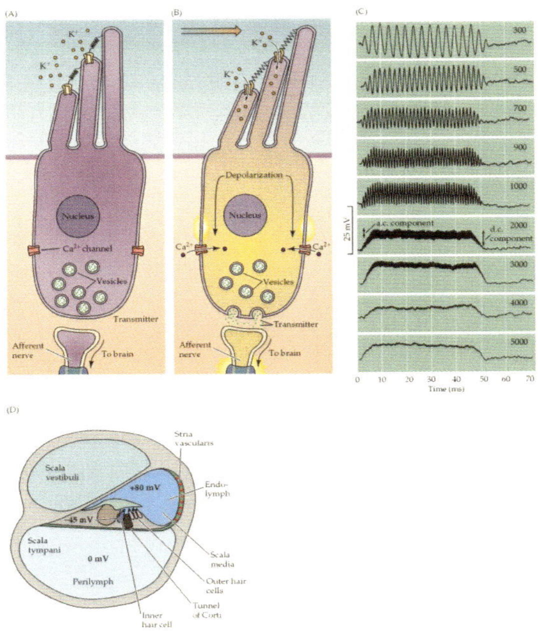

Mechanoelectrical transduction mediated by hair cells. (A,B) When the hair bundle is deflected toward the tallest stereocilium, cation-selective channels open near the tips of the stereocilia, allowing K^+ ions to flow into the hair cell down their electrochemical gradient (see text on next page for the explanation of this peculiar situation). The resulting depolarization of the hair cell opens voltage-gated Ca^{2+} channels in the cell soma, allowing calcium entry and release of neurotransmitter onto the nerve endings of the auditory nerve. (C) Receptor potentials generated by an individual hair cell in the cochlea in response to pure tones (indicated in Hz at the right of the tracings). Note that the hair cell potential faithfully follows the waveform of the stimulating sinusoids for low frequencies (<3kHz), but still responds with a DC offset to higher frequencies. (D) The stereocilia of the hair cells protrude into the endolymph, which is high in K^+ and has an electrical potential of +80 mV relative to the perilymph.

Understanding the ionic basis of hair cell transduction has been greatly advanced by intracellular recordings made from these tiny structures. The hair cell has a resting potential between -45 and -60 mV relative to the fluid that bathes the basal end of the cell. At the resting potential, only a small fraction of the transduction channels are open. When the hair bundle is displaced in the direction of the tallest stereocilium, more transduction channels open, causing depolarization as K^+ enters the cell. Depolarization in turn opens voltage-gated calcium channels in the hair cell membrane, and the resultant Ca^{2+} influx causes transmitter release from the basal end of the cell onto the auditory nerve endings . Such calcium-dependent exocytosis is similar to chemical neurotransmission elsewhere in the central and peripheral nervous system . Because some of the transduction channels are open at rest, the receptor potential is biphasic: Movement toward the tallest stereocilia depolarizes the cell, while movement in the opposite direction leads to hyperpolarization. This situation allows the hair cell to generate a sinusoidal receptor potential in response to a sinusoidal stimulus, thus preserving the temporal information present in the original signal up to frequencies of around 3 kHz.

Inner Hair Cells – From Sound to Nerve Signal

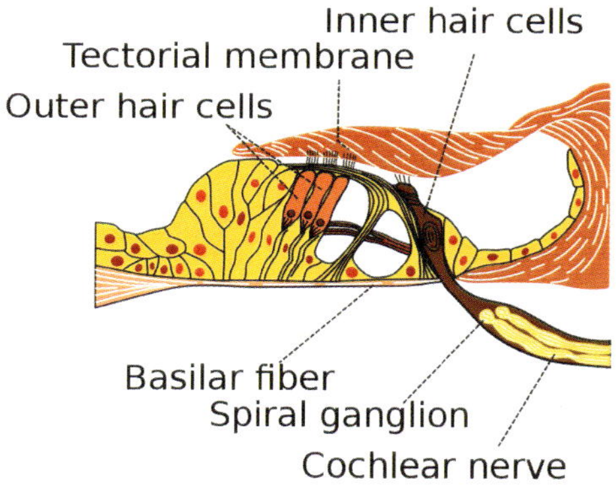

Section through the organ of Corti, showing inner and outer hair cells

The deflection of the hair-cell stereocilia opens mechanically gated ion channels that allow any small, positively charged ions (primarily potassium and calcium) to enter the cell. Unlike many other electrically active cells, the hair cell itself does not fire an action potential. Instead, the influx of positive ions from the endolymph in the scala media depolarizes the cell, resulting in a receptor potential. This receptor potential opens voltage gated calcium channels; calcium ions then enter the cell and trigger the release of neurotransmitters at the basal end of the cell. The neurotransmitters diffuse across the narrow space between the hair cell and a nerve terminal, where they then bind to receptors and thus trigger action potentials in the nerve. In this way, the mechanical sound signal is converted into an electrical nerve signal. Repolarization of hair cells is done in a special manner. The perilymph in the scala tympani has a very low concentration of positive ions. The electrochemical gradient makes the positive ions flow through channels to the perilymph.

Hair cells chronically leak Ca^{2+}. This leakage causes a tonic release of neurotransmitter to the synapses. It is thought that this tonic release is what allows the hair cells to respond so quickly in response to mechanical stimuli. The quickness of the hair cell response may also be due to the fact that it can increase the amount of neurotransmitter release in response to a change as little as 100 μV in membrane potential.

Outer Hair Cells – Acoustical Pre-amplifiers

In mammalian outer hair cells, the receptor potential triggers active vibrations of the cell body. This mechanical response to electrical signals is termed somatic electromotility and drives oscillations in the cell's length, which occur at the frequency of the incoming sound and provide mechanical feedback amplification. Outer hair cells are found only in mammals. While hearing sensitivity of mammals is similar to that of other classes of vertebrates, without functioning outer hair cells, the sensitivity decreases by approximately 50 dB. Outer hair cells extend the hearing range to about 200 kHz in some marine mammals. They have also improved frequency selectivity (frequency discrimination), which is of particular benefit for humans, because it enabled sophisticated speech and music.

The effect of this system is to non-linearly amplify quiet sounds more than large ones so that a wide range of sound pressures can be reduced to a much smaller range of hair displacements. This property of amplification is called the cochlear amplifier.

The molecular biology of hair cells has seen considerable progress in recent years, with the identification of the motor protein (prestin) that underlies somatic electromotility in the outer hair cells. Prestin's function has been shown to be dependent on chloride channel signaling and that it is compromised by the common marine pesticide tributyltin. Because this class of pollutant bioconcentrates up the food chain, the effect is pronounced in top marine predators such as orcas and toothed whales.

Hair Cell Signal Adaption

Calcium ion influx plays an important role for the hair cells to adapt to the amplification of the signal. This allows humans to ignore constant sounds that are no longer new and allow us to be acute to other changes in our surrounding. The key adaptation mechanism comes from a motor protein myosin-1c that allows slow adaptation, provides tension to sensitize transduction channels, and also participate in signal transduction apparatus. More recent research now shows that the calcium-sensitive binding of calmodulin to myosin-1c could actually modulate the interaction of the adaptation motor with other components of the transduction apparatus as well.

Fast Adaptation: During fast adaptation, Ca^{2+}ions that enter a stereocilium through an open MET channel bind rapidly to a site on or near the channel and induce channel closure. When channels close, tension increases in the tip link, pulling the bundle in the opposite direction. Fast adaptation is more prominent in sound and auditory detecting hair cells, rather in vestibular cells.

Slow Adaption: The dominating model suggests that slow adaptation occurs when myosin-1c slides down the stereocilium in response to elevated tension during bundle displacement. The resultant decreased tension in the tip link permits the bundle to move farther in the opposite direction. As tension decreases, channels close, producing the decline in transduction current. Slow adaptation is most prominent in vestibular hair cells that sense spatial movement and less in cochlear hair cells that detect auditory signals.

Neuronal Encoding of Sound

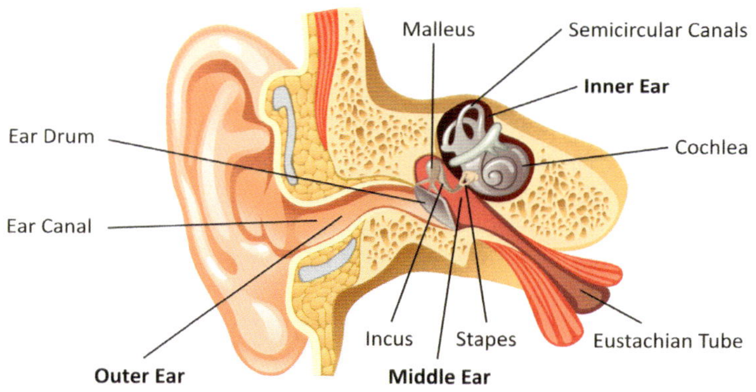

There are three main sections of our hearing system: the outer ear, the middle ear, and the inner ear (please image above). Each section of the ear plays a role in the way we perceive sound.

First Step: Sound waves travel through the outer ear. Once the waves reach the end of the ear canal the ear drum begins to vibrate transforming the sound wave energy into mechanical energy.

Second Step: The vibration of the ear drum initiates movement of the three ear bones. These bones are called the malleus, incus and stapes. The malleus, which is directly attached to the ear drum, immediately moves in response to the vibrations. This motion in turn moves the incus which triggers the activation of the stapes.

Third Step: The stapes then transmits the mechanical energy (carried by the bones) into the inner ear in the form of hydraulic energy. The stapes collides with the cochlea which sends a wave of fluid moving across the cochlea's membrane. This fluid stimulates the hair cells on the membrane of the cochlea, where the hair cells convert the hydraulic energy into electric energy.

Fourth Step: The auditory nerve is stimulated by the hair cells, which in turn conducts the signals to the brain for further processing. The brain is able to processes sound by determining where in the cochlea the signal originates. The base of the cochlea (where the stapes collides) is responsible for higher frequency where the apex (the farthest point from the stapes) is responsible for lower frequency sounds.

Wave Properties

We are not going to go into too much detail about the wave's physical properties, since it is out of the scope of this atom, but remember:

- Frequency is perceived by humans as pitch;
- The sound intensity is the amplitude;
- Humans can only hear a specific range of sound, usually from 20 Hz to 20,000 Hz;
- The factors that go into a sound are its intensity, frequency and overtones (which are like interference, or background noises).

The complexities of contemporary neuroscience are continually redefined. Thus what is known now of the auditory system has changed in the recent times and thus conceivably in the next two years or so, much of this will change.

This article is structured in a format that starts with a small exploration of what sound is followed by the general anatomy of the ear which in turn will finally give way to explaining the encoding mechanism of the engineering marvel that is the ear. This article traces the route that sound waves first take from generation at an unknown source to their integration and perception by the auditory cortex.

Basic Physics of Sound

Sound waves are what physicists call longitudinal waves, which consist of propagating regions of high pressure (compression) and corresponding regions of low pressure (rarefaction).

Waveform

Waveform is a description of the general shape of the sound wave. Waveforms are sometimes described by the sum of sinusoids, via Fourier analysis.

Amplitude

Amplitude is the size of the pressure variations in a sound wave, and primarily determines the loudness with which the sound is perceived. In a sinusoidal function such as $C\sin(2\pi ft)$, C represents the amplitude of the sound wave.

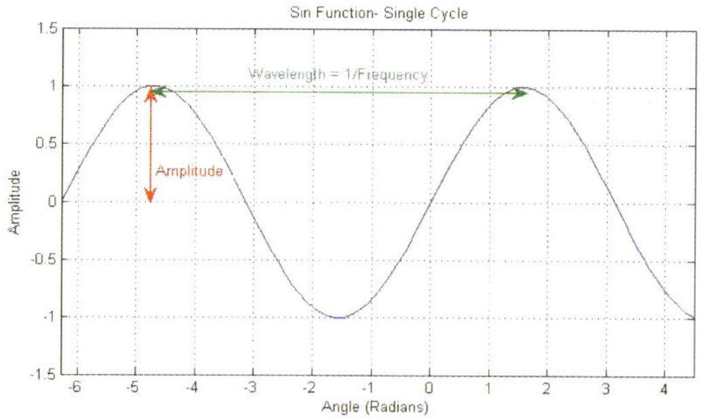

Graph of a simple sine wave

Frequency and Wavelength

The frequency of a sound is defined as the number of repetitions of its waveform per second, and is measured in hertz; frequency is inversely proportional to wavelength (in a medium of uniform propagation velocity, such as sound in air). The wavelength of a sound is the distance between any two consecutive matching points on the waveform. The audible frequency range for young humans is about 20 Hz to 20 kHz. Hearing of higher frequencies decreases with age, limiting to about 16 kHz for adults, and even down to 3 kHz for elders.

Anatomy of the Ear

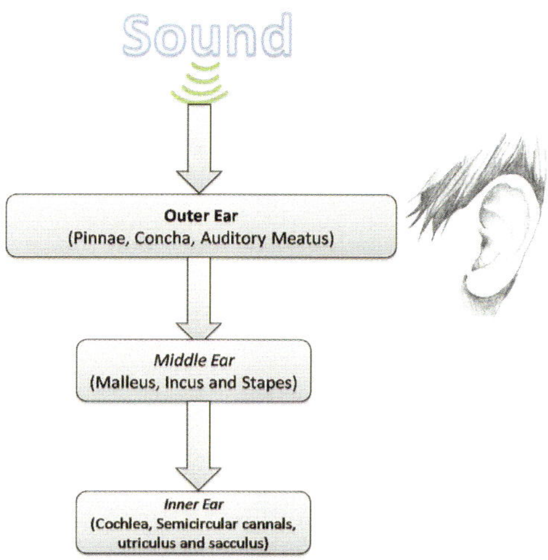

Flowchart of sound passage - outer ear

Given the simple physics of sound, the anatomy and physiology of hearing can be studied in greater detail.

Outer Ear

The Outer ear consists of the pinna or auricle (visible parts including ear lobes and concha), and the auditory meatus (the passageway for sound). The fundamental function of this part of the ear is to gather sound energy and deliver it to the eardrum. Resonances of the external ear selectively boost sound pressure with frequency in the range 2–5 kHz.

The pinna as a result of its asymmetrical structure is able to provide further cues about the elevation from which the sound originated. The vertical asymmetry of the pinna selectively amplifies sounds of higher frequency from high elevation thereby providing spatial information by virtue of its mechanical design.

Middle Ear

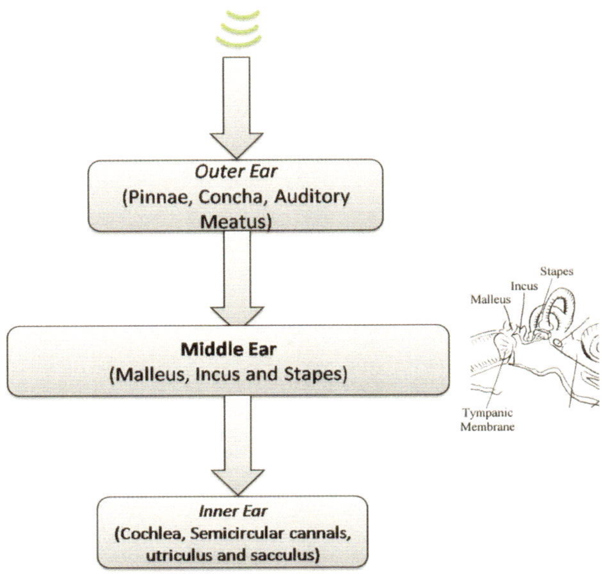

Flowchart of sound passage - middle ear

The middle ear plays a crucial role in the auditory process, as it essentially converts pressure variations in air to perturbations in the fluids of the inner ear. In other words, it is the mechanical transfer function that allows for efficient transfer of collected sound energy between two different media. The three small bones that are responsible for this complex process are the malleus, the incus, and the stapes, collectively known as the ear ossicles. The impedance matching is done through via lever ratios and the ratio of areas of the tympanic membrane and the footplate of the stapes, creating a transformer-like mechanism. Furthermore, the ossicles are arranged in such a manner as to resonate at 700–800 Hz while at the same time protecting the inner ear from excessive energy. A certain degree of top-down control is present at the middle ear level primarily through two muscles present in this anatomical region: the tensor tympani and the stapedius. These two muscles can restrain the ossicles so as to reduce the amount of energy that is transmitted into the inner ear in loud surroundings.

Inner Ear

The cochlea of the inner ear, a marvel of physiological engineering, acts as both a frequency analyzer and nonlinear acoustic amplifier. The cochlea has over 32,000 hair cells. Outer hair cells primarily provide amplification of traveling waves that are induced by sound energy, while inner hair cells detect the motion of those waves and excite the (Type I) neurons of the auditory nerve.

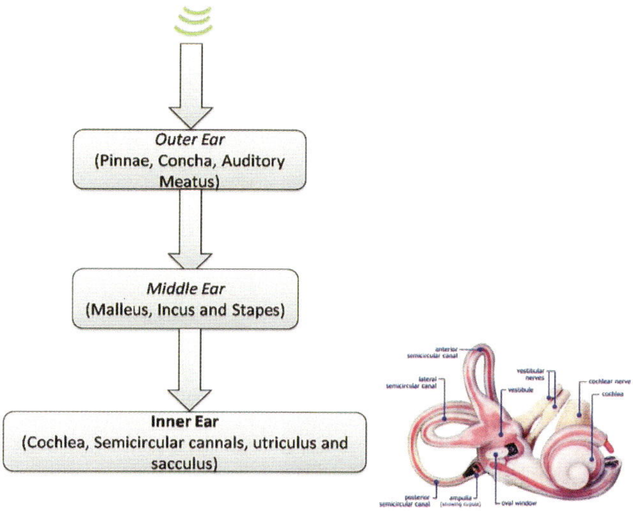

Flowchart of sound passage - inner ear

The basal end of the cochlea, where sounds enter from the middle ear, encodes the higher end of the audible frequency range while the apical end of the cochlea encodes the lower end of the frequency range. This tonotopy plays a crucial role in hearing, as it allows for spectral separation of sounds. A cross section of the cochlea will reveal an anatomical structure with three main chambers (scala vestibuli, scala media, and scala tympani). At the apical end of the cochlea, at an opening known as the helicotrema, the scala vestibuli merges with the scala tympani. The fluid found in these two cochlear chambers is perilymph, while scala media, or the cochlear duct, is filled with endolymph.

Transduction

Auditory Hair Cells

The auditory hair cells in the cochlea are at the core of the auditory system's special functionality (similar hair cells are located in the semicircular canals). Their primary function is mechanotransduction, or conversion between mechanical and neural signals. The relatively small number of the auditory hair cells is surprising when compared to other sensory cells such as the rods and cones of the visual system. Thus the loss of a lower number (in the order of thousands) of auditory hair cells can be devastating while the loss of a larger number of retinal cells (in the order to hundreds of thousands) will not be as bad from a sensory standpoint.

Cochlear hair cells are organized as inner hair cells and outer hair cells; inner and outer refer to relative position from the axis of the cochlear spiral. The inner hair cells are the primary sensory receptors and a significant amount of the sensory input to the auditory cortex occurs from these hair cells. Outer hair cells on the other hand boost the mechanical signal by using electromechanical feedback.

Mechanotransduction

The apical surface of each cochlear hair cell contains a hair bundle. Each hair bundle contains approximately 300 fine projections known as stereocilia, formed by actin cytoskeletal elements. The stereocilia in a hair bundle are arranged in multiple rows of different heights. In addition to the stereocilia, a true ciliary structure known as the kinocilium exists and is believed to play a role in hair cell degeneration that is caused by exposure to high frequencies.

A stereocilium is able to bend at its point of attachment to the apical surface of the hair cell. The actin filaments that form the core of a stereocilium are highly interlinked and cross linked with fibrin, and are therefore stiff and inflexible at positions other than the base. When stereocilia in the tallest row are deflected in the positive-stimulus direction, the shorter rows of stereocilia are also deflected. These simultaneous deflections occur due to filaments called tip links that attach the side of each taller stereocilium to the top of the shorter stereocilium in the adjacent row. When the tallest stereocilia are deflected, tension is produced in the tip links and causes the stereocilia in the other rows to deflect as well. At the lower end of each tip link is one or more mechano-electrical transduction (MET) channels, which are opened by tension in the tip links. These MET channels are cation-selective transduction channels that allow potassium and calcium ions to enter the hair cell from the endolymph that bathes its apical end.

The influx of cations, particularly potassium, through the open MET channels causes the membrane potential of the hair cell to depolarize. This depolarization opens voltage-gated calcium channels to allow the further influx of calcium. This results in an increase in the calcium concentration, which triggers the exocytosis of neurotransmitter vesicles at ribbon synapses at the basolateral surface of the hair cell. The release of neurotransmitter at a ribbon synapse, in turn, generates an action potential in the connected auditory-nerve fiber. Hyperpolarization of the hair cell, which occurs when potassium leaves the cell, is also important, as it stops the influx of calcium and therefore stops the fusion of vesicles at the ribbon synapses. Thus, as elsewhere in the body, the transduction is dependent on the concentration and distribution of ions. The perilymph that is found in the scala tympani has a low potassium concentration, whereas the endolymph found in the scala media has a high potassium concentration and an electrical potential of about 80 millivolts compared to the perilymph. Mechanotransduction by stereocilia is highly sensitive and able to detect perturbations as small as fluid fluctuations of 0.3 nanometers, and can convert this mechanical stimulation into an electrical nerve impulse in about 10 microseconds.

Nerve Fibers from the Cochlea

There are two types of afferent neurons found in the cochlear nerve: Type I and Type II. Each type of neuron has specific cell selectivity within the cochlea. The mechanism that determines the selectivity of each type of neuron for a specific hair cell has been proposed by two diametrically opposed theories in neuroscience known as the peripheral instruction hypothesis and the cell autonomous instruction hypothesis. The peripheral instruction hypothesis states that phenotypic differentiation between the two neurons are not made until after these undifferentiated neurons attach to hair cells which in turn will dictate the differentiation pathway. The cell autonomous instruction hypothesis states that differentiation into Type I and Type II neurons occur following the last phase of mitotic division but preceding innervations. Both types of neuron participate in the encoding of sound for transmission to the brain.

Type I Neurons

Type I neurons innervate inner hair cells. There is significantly greater convergence of this type of neuron towards the basal end in comparison with the apical end. A radial fiber bundle acts as an intermediary between Type I neurons and inner hair cells. The ratio of innervation that is seen between Type I neurons and inner hair cells is 1:1 which results in high signal transmission fidelity and resolution.

Type II Neurons

Type II neurons on the other hand innervate outer hair cells. However, there is significantly greater convergence of this type of neuron towards the apex end in comparison with the basal end. A 1:30-60 ratio of innervation is seen between Type II neurons and outer hair cells which in turn make these neurons ideal for electromechanical feedback. Type II neurons can be physiologically manipulated to innervate inner hair cells provided outer hair cells have been destroyed either through mechanical damage or by chemical damage induced by drugs such as gentamicin.

Auditory Cortex

Primary auditory neurons carry action potentials from the cochlea into the transmission pathway shown in the adjacent image. Multiple relay stations act as integration and processing centers. The signals reach the first level of cortical processing at the primary auditory cortex (A1), in the superior temporal gyrus of the temporal lobe. Most areas up to and including A1 are tonotopically mapped (that is, frequencies are kept in an ordered arrangement). However, A1 participates in coding more complex and abstract aspects of auditory stimuli without coding well the frequency content, including the presence of a distinct sound or its echoes. Like lower regions, this region of the brain has combination-sensitive neurons that have nonlinear responses to stimuli.

Recent studies conducted in bats and other mammals have revealed that the ability to process and interpret modulation in frequencies primarily occurs in the superior and middle temporal gyri of the temporal lobe. Lateralization of brain function exists in the cortex, with the processing of speech in the left cerebral hemisphere and environmental sounds in the right hemisphere of the auditory cortex. Music, with its influence on emotions, is also processed in the right hemisphere of the auditory cortex. While the reason for such localization is not quite understood, lateralization in this instance does not imply exclusivity as both hemispheres do participate in the processing, but one hemisphere tends to play a more significant role than the other.

Neuronal Structure

Cochlear Nucleus

The cochlear nuclei (CN) in man consist of the dorsal (DCN), superior ventral (SVCN), and inferior ventral (IVCN). The CN is located on the dorsolateral surface of the brain stem at the junction of the medulla with the pons.

The posterior cochlear nucleus and the anterior cochlear nucleus are located lateral and posterior to the restiform body and are partially on the surface of the brainstem at the pontomedullary junction. The posterior cochlear nucleus drapes over the restiform body just inferior to the pontomedullary junction. At this level, the posterior part of the anterior cochlear nucleus is small in proportion to the posterior cochlear nucleus . The anterior cochlear nucleus extends rostral to the posterior cochlear nucleus , where it may be covered by the flocculus and by caudal fascicles of the middle cerebellar peduncle.

All cochlear nerve fibers end in the cochlear nuclei on the ipsilateral side. As these fibers enter the brainstem at the cerebellopontine angle, they divide into ascending and descending bundles. Fibers in the ascending bundle synapse in the anterior part of the anterior cochlear nucleus, whereas fibers in the descending bundle synapse in the posterior part of the anterior cochlear nucleus and in the posterior cochlear nucleus.

In the cochlear nuclei, each afferent nerve fiber makes specialized synaptic contacts with several different cell types. Individual fibers and their synaptic contacts distribute along orderly rows so that the resulting order produces distinct tonotopic maps in each division.

Specific cell types of the cochlear nuclei, in turn, give rise to parallel but separate ascending pathways in the auditory system that analyze and code different sound features while preserving frequency information. These projections are subdivided into pathways conveying monaural information to the inferior colliculus and those providing input to the superior olivary complex for binaural processing. Most fibers from the anterior cochlear nucleus course anterior to the restiform body part of the inferior cerebellar peduncle to form the trapezoid body. Projections from the posterior cochlear nucleus and some from the anterior cochlear nucleus course posteriorly over the restiform body as the posterior acoustic stria and decussate in the pontine tegmentum before joining the lateral lemniscus.

The auditory nerve penetrates through the skull and forms a first relay station at the level of the cochlear nuclei.

Nerve fibers entering the cochlear nuclei are distributed in an organised, tonotopic, manner: those that come from the apex of the cochlea (low frequencies) remain at the surface of the cochlear nuclei, whereas those of the base (high frequencies) penetrate deeper into the nuclei. This distribution allows each frequency to activate neurones located in a band that is sensitive to stimulation from a specific frequency known as isofrequency laminae.

Each fiber divides into a "V" shape with two branches: one ventral ascending (for the ventral nucleus) and another dorsal-descending (for the posterior and dorsal cochlear nuclei).

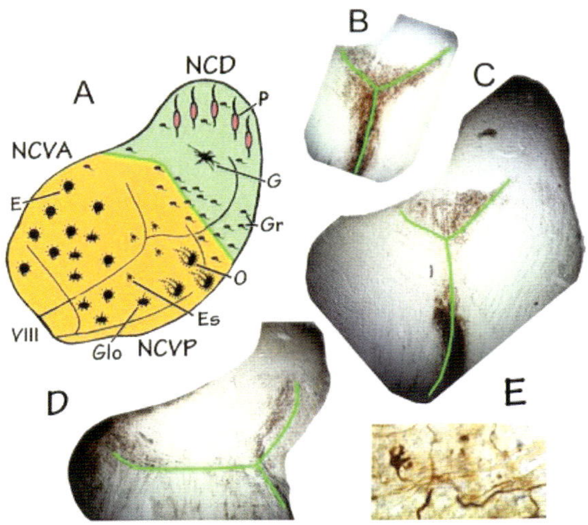

In this diagram, you can see the tonotopic 'V'

- DCN = Dorsal cochlear nucleus
- AVCN = anterior ventral cochlear nucleus
- PVCN = posterior ventral cochlear nucleus

Types de neurones: Neural types:

- E = Spherical bushy
- Glo = Globular cells
- Es = Stellate cells
- O = Octopus cells
- Gr = Granular cells
- G = Giant cells
- PF = fusiform and pyramidal cells

Function

The cochlear nuclei decode intensity, analyse various temporal parameters such as duration (long or short sounds) and the start and end of a sound stimulus, and maintain and transmit the frequency analysis carried out previously at the level of the cochlea.

The function of each type of neuron is well defined. They have the essential role of completing the frequency and intensity analyses started at the cochlea.

- Globular and spherical neurons have a primary response similar to that of the spiral ganglion. neurons: they respond continuously throughout a stimulus.
- Octopus cells fire at the beginning of the stimulus ('onset response').
- Fusiform and pyramidal cells of the DCN fire at the beginning of the stimulus ('on-off' response).

The cochlear nuclei have numerous internal circuits with excitatory or inhibitory connections between neurons, which contribute to the analysis of the auditory signal and its distribution towards the higher centres of the auditory system, starting with the the next relay centre: the superior olivary complex.

Projections to the Cochlear Nuclei

The major input to the cochlear nucleus is from the auditory nerve, a part of cranial nerve VIII (the vestibulocochlear nerve). The auditory nerve fibers form a highly organized system of connections according to their peripheral innervation of the cochlea. Axons from the spiral ganglion cells of the lower frequencies innervate the ventrolateral portions of the ventral cochlear nucleus and lateral-ventral portions of the dorsal cochlear nucleus. The axons from the higher frequency organ of corti hair cells project to the dorsal portion of the ventral cochlear nucleus and the dorsal-medial portions of the dorsal cochlear nucleus. The mid frequency projections end up in between the two extremes; in this way the tonotopic organization that is established in the cochlea is preserved in the cochlear nuclei. This tonotopic organization is preserved because only a few inner hair cells synapse on the dendrites of a nerve cell in the spiral ganglion, and the axon from that nerve cell synapses on only a very few dendrites in the cochlear nucleus. In contrast with the VCN that receives all acoustic input from the auditory nerve, the DCN receives input not only from the auditory nerve but it also receives acoustic input from neurons in the VCN (T stellate cells). The DCN is therefore in a sense a second order sensory nucleus.

The cochlear nuclei have long been thought to receive input only from the ipsilateral ear. There is evidence, however, for stimulation from the contralateral ear via the contralateral CN, and also the somatosensory parts of the brain.

Projections from the Cochlear Nuclei

There are three major fiber bundles, axons of cochlear nuclear neurons, that carry information from the cochlear nuclei to targets that are mainly on the opposite side of the brain. Through the medulla, one projection goes to the contralateral superior olivary complex (SOC) via the trapezoid body, whilst the other half shoots to the ipsilateral SOC. This pathway is called the ventral acoustic stria (VAS or, more commonly, the trapezoid body). Another pathway, called the dorsal acoustic stria (DAS, also known as the stria of von Monakow), rises above the medulla into the pons where it hits the nuclei of the lateral lemniscus along with its kin, the intermediate acoustic stria (IAS, also known as the stria of Held). The IAS decussates across the medulla, before joining the ascending fibers in the contralateral lateral lemniscus. The lateral lemniscus contains cells of the nuclei of the lateral lemniscus, and in turn projects to the inferior colliculus. The inferior colliculus receives direct, monosynaptic projections from the superior olivary complex the contralateral dorsal acoustic stria, some classes of stellate neurons of the VCN, as well as from the different nuclei of the lateral lemniscus.

Most of these inputs terminate in the inferior colliculus, although there are a few small projections that bypass the inferior colliculus and project to the medial geniculate, or other forebrain structures.

- Medial superior olive (MSO) via trapezoid body (TB) – Ipsilateral and contralateral stimulation for low frequency sounds.
- Lateral superior olive (LSO) directly and via TB – Ipsilateral stimulation for high frequency sounds.
- Medial nucleus of trapezoid body (MNTB) – Contralateral stimulation.
- Inferior colliculus – Contralateral stimulation.
- Periolivary nuclei (PON) – Ipsilateral and contralateral stimulation.

- Lateral lemniscus (LL) and lemniscal nuclei (LN) – Ipsilateral and contralateral stimulation.

Histology

Three types of principal cells convey information out of the ventral cochlear nucleus: Bushy cells, stellate cells, and octopus cells.

- *Bushy cells* are found mainly in the anterior ventral cochlear nucleus (AVCN). These can be further divided into large spherical, small spherical and globular bushy cells, depending on their appearance, and also their location. Within the AVCN there is an area of large spherical cells; caudal to this are smaller spherical cells, and globular cells occupy the region around the nerve root. An important difference between these subtypes is that they project to differing targets in the superior olivary complex. Large spherical bushy cells project to the ipsilateral and contralateral medial superior olive. Globular bushy cells project to the contralateral medial nucleus of the trapezoid body, and small spherical bushy cells likely project to the lateral superior olive. They have a few (1-4) very short dendrites with numerous small branching, which cause it to resemble a "bush". The bushy cells have specialized electrical properties that allow them to transmit timing information from the auditory nerve to more central areas of the auditory system. Because bushy cells receive input from multiple auditory nerve fibers that are tuned to similar frequencies, bushy cells can improve the precision of the timing information by in essence averaging out jitter in timing of the inputs. Bushy cells can also be inhibited by sounds adjacent to the frequency to which they are tuned, leading to even sharper tuning than seen in auditory nerve fibers. These cells are usually innervated only by a few auditory nerve fibres, which dominate its firing pattern. These afferent nerve fibres wrap their terminal branches around the entire soma, creating a large synapse onto the bushy cells, called an "endbulb of Held". Therefore, a single unit recording of an electrically stimulated bushy neuron characteristically produces exactly one action potential and constitutes the primary response.

- *Stellate cells* (aka multipolar cells), have longer dendrites that lie parallel to fascicles of auditory nerve fibers. They are also called chopper cells, in reference to their ability to fire a regularly spaced train of action potentials for the duration of a tonal or noise stimulus. The chopping pattern is intrinsic to the electrical excitability of the stellate cell, and the firing rate depends on the strength of the auditory input more than on the frequency. Each stellate cell is narrowly tuned and has inhibitory sidebands, enabling the population of stellate cells to encode the spectrum of sounds, enhancing spectral peaks and valleys. These neurons provide acoustic input to the DCN.

- *Octopus cells* are found in a small region of the posterior ventral cochlear nucleus (PVCN). The distinguishing features of these cells are their long, thick and tentacle-shaped dendrites that typically emanate from one side of the cell body. Octopus cells produce an "Onset Response" to simple tonal stimuli. That is, they respond only at the onset of a broad-band stimulus. The octopus cells can fire with some of the highest temporal precision of any neuron in the brain. Electrical stimuli to the auditory nerve evoke a graded excitatory postsynaptic potential in the octopus cells. These EPSPs are very brief. The octopus cells are thought to be important for extracting timing information. It has been reported that these cells can respond to click trains at a rate of 800 Hz.

Two types of principal cells convey information out of the dorsal cochlear nucleus (DCN) to the contralateral inferior colliculus. The principal cells receive two systems of inputs. Acoustic input comes to the deep layer through several paths. Excitatory acoustic input comes from auditory nerve fibers and also from stellate cells of the VCN. Acoustic input is also conveyed through inhibitory interneurons (tuberculoventral cells of the DCN and "wide band inhibitors" in the VCN). Through the outermost molecular layer, the DCN receives other types of sensory information, most importantly information about the location of the head and ears, through parallel fibers. This information is distributed through a cerebellar like circuit that also includes inhibitory interneurons.

- *Fusiform cells* (also known as *pyramidal cells*). Fusiform cells integrate information through two tufts of dendrites, the apical dendrites receiving multisensory, excitatory and inhibitory input through the outermost molecular layer and the basal dendrites receiving excitatory and inhibitory acoustic input from the basal dendrites that extend into the deep layer. These neurons are thought to enable mammals to analyze the spectral cues that enable us to localize sounds in elevation and when we lose hearing in one ear.

- *Giant cells* also integrate inputs from the molecular and deep layers but input from the deep layer is predominant. It is unclear what their role is in hearing.

Function

The cochlear nuclear complex is the first integrative, or processing, stage in the auditory system. Information is brought to the nuclei from the ipsilateral cochlea via the cochlear nerve. Several tasks are performed in the cochlear nuclei. By distributing acoustic input to multiple types of principal cells, the auditory pathway is subdivided into parallel ascending pathways, which can simultaneously extract different types of information. The cells of the ventral cochlear nucleus extract information that is carried by the auditory nerve in the timing of firing and in the pattern of activation of the population of auditory nerve fibers. The cells of the dorsal cochlear nucleus perform a non-linear spectral analysis and place that spectral analysis into the context of the location of the head, ears and shoulders and that separate expected, self-generated spectral cues from more interesting, unexpected spectral cues using input from the auditory cortex, pontine nuclei, trigeminal ganglion and nucleus, dorsal column nuclei and the second dorsal root ganglion. It is likely that these neurons help mammals to use spectral cues for orienting toward those sounds. The information is used by higher brainstem regions to achieve further computational objectives (such as sound source location or improvement in signal to noise ratio). The inputs from these other areas of the brain probably play a role in sound localization.

In order to understand in more detail the specific functions of the cochlear nuclei it is first necessary to understand the way sound information is represented by the fibers of the auditory nerve. Briefly, there are around 30,000 auditory nerve fibres in each of the two auditory nerves. Each fiber is an axon of a spiral ganglion cell that represents a particular frequency of sound, and a particular range of loudness. Information in each nerve fibre is represented by the rate of action potentials as well as the particular timing of individual action potentials. The particular physiology and morphology of each cochlear nucleus cell type enhances different aspects of sound information.

Ventral Cochlear Nucleus

In the ventral cochlear nucleus (VCN), auditory nerve fibers enter the brain via the nerve root in the VCN. The ventral cochlear nucleus is divided into the anterior ventral (anteroventral) cochlear nucleus (AVCN) and the posterior ventral (posteroventral) cochlear nucleus (PVCN). In the VCN, auditory nerve fibers bifurcate, the ascending branch innervates the AVCN and the descending branch innervates the PVCN and then continue to the dorsal cochlear nucleus. The orderly innervation by auditory nerve fibers gives the AVCN a tonotopic organization along the dorsoventral axis. Fibers that carry information from the apex of the cochlea that are tuned to low frequencies contact neurons in the ventral part of the AVCN; those that carry information from the base of the cochlea that are tuned to high frequencies contact neurons in the dorsal part of the AVCN. Several populations of neurons populate the AVCN. Bushy cells receive input from auditory nerve fibers through particularly large endings called end bulbs of Held. They contact stellate cells through more conventional boutons.

Cell Types

The anterior cochlear nucleus contains several cell types, which correspond fairly well with different physiological unit types. Additionally, these cell types generally have specific projection patterns.

Bushy Cells

Named due to the branching, tree-like, nature of their dendritic fields, visible using Golgi's method, they receive large end bulbs of Held from auditory nerve fibers. Bushy cells are of three subtypes that project to different target nuclei in the superior olivary complex.

Globular

Globular bushy cells project large axons to the contralateral medial nucleus of the trapezoid body (MNTB), in the superior olivary complex where they synapse onto principal cells via a single calyx of Held, and several smaller collaterals synapse ipsilaterally in the posterior (PPO) and dorsolateral periolivary (DLPO) nuclei, lateral superior olive (LSO), and lateral nucleus of the trapezoid body (LNTB); contralaterally in the dorsomedial periolivary nucleus (DMPO), ventral nucleus of the trapezoid body (VNTB), nucleus paragigantocellularis lateralis (PGL), and ventral nucleus of the lateral lemniscus (VNLL). Axons always send a collateral into the MNTB, but do not necessarily give rise to collaterals that innervate each of the other nuclei.

Large Spherical

Spherical bushy cells project ipsilaterally to the LSO, bilaterally to the medial superior olive (MSO) and LNTB, and contralaterally to the VNTB and VNLL. The most important purpose of these projections seems to be to imbue the MSO and LSO with their interaural time and level sensitivities (respectively).

Small Spherical

Small spherical bushy cells likely project to the ipsilateral lateral superior olive. They project neither to the medial superior olives or to the medial nucleus of the trapezoid body.

Multipolar Cells

Multipolar cells fall into two distinct groups. Those whose axons project out of the aVCN through the trapezoid body, T stellate cells, have longer dendrites than bushy cells that characteristically lie in line with fascicles of auditory nerve fibers. These principal cells are excitatory.

Another name for these cells is 'choppers'. They have an intrinsical rhythm, and will fire action potentials with this rhythm once activated by the right sound.

Anterior Ventral Cochlear Nucleus (AVCN)

The anteroventral cochlear nucleus (AVCN) (or accessory), is placed between the two divisions of the cochlear nerve, and is on the ventral aspect of the inferior peduncle.

- The AVCN can be subdivided based upon the cytoarchitecture of the region.
    - Typical subdivisions are defined as: anterior (AaVCN), posterior (PaVCN), posterodorsal (PDaVCN), and posteroventral (PVaVCN).
- A well-defined tonotopy is evident. Lateral PVaVCN, medial PVaVCN, and

medial PDaVCN roughly correspond to the low (<1 kHz), middle (4–8 kHz), and high (>16 kHz) frequency regions defined by Bourk.

- The aVCN projects to nearly all brainstem auditory structures. High frequency regions tend to project contralaterally, and low frequency regions bilaterally, preserving the tonotopic organization of the ascending auditory pathway.
- Stellate/multipolar cells form the projection to both inferior colliculi (central nucleus and dorsal cortex), and synapse in a banded pattern, following the tonotopy of the region.

Dorsal Cochlear Nucleus

The dorsal cochlear nucleus (DCN, also known as the "tuberculum acusticum"), is a cortex-like structure on the dorso-lateral surface of the brainstem. Along with the ventral cochlear nucleus (VCN), it forms the cochlear nucleus (CN), where all auditory nerve fibers from the cochlea form their first synapses.

Anatomy

The DCN differs from the ventral portion of the CN as it not only projects to the central nucleus (a subdivision) of the inferior colliculus (CIC), but also receives efferent innervation from the auditory cortex, superior olivary complex and the inferior colliculus. The cytoarchitecture and neurochemistry of the DCN is similar to that of the cerebellum, a concept that currently is important in theories of DCN function. Thus, the DCN is thought to be involved with more complex auditory processing, rather than merely transferring information.

The pyramidal cells or giant cells are a major cell grouping of the DCN. These cells are the target of two different input systems. The first system arises from the auditory nerve, and carries acoustic information. The second set of inputs is relayed through a set of small granule cells in the cochlear nucleus. There are also a great number of neighbouring cartwheel cells. The granule cells in turn are the target of a number of different inputs, including both those involved in auditory processing and, at least in lower mammals, somatosensory inputs associated with the head, the ear, and the jaw.

Projections from DCN principal cells form the dorsal acoustic stria, which ultimately terminate in the CIC. This projection overlaps with that of the lateral superior olive (LSO) in a well-defined manner, where they form the primary excitatory input for ICC type O units.

Physiology

Principal cells in the DCN have very complex frequency intensity tuning curves. Classified as cochlear nucleus type IV cells, the firing rate may be very rapid in response to a low intensity sound at one frequency and then fall below the spontaneous rate with only a small increment in stimulus frequency or intensity. The firing rate may then increase with another increment in intensity or frequency. Type IV cells are excited by wide band noise, and particularly excited by a noise-notch stimulus directly below the cell's best frequency (BF).

While the VCN bushy cells aid in the location of a sound stimulus on the horizontal axis via their inputs to the superior olivary complex, type IV cells may participate in localization of the sound stimulus on the vertical axis. The pinna selectively amplifies frequencies, resulting in reduced sound energy at specific frequencies in certain regions of space. The complicated firing patterns of type IV cells makes them especially suited to detecting these notches, and with the combined power of these two localization systems, an ordinary person can locate where a firework explodes without the use of their eyes.

Somatosensory inputs inhibit type IV cell activity, possibly silencing their activity during head and pinna movements. While this has not been studied extensively, it may play an important role in sound source localization in elevation. A similar effect is seen in the visual system in an effect known as change blindness.

Current auditory models of the DCN employ a two-inhibitor model. Type IV cells receive excitation directly from the auditory nerve, and are inhibited by type II (vertical) cells and a wide band inhibitor (onset-c cells).

Trapezoid Body

The medial nucleus of the trapezoid body (MNTB) is a collection of brainstem neurons that function within the ascending auditory pathway. MNTB neurons are associated with a number of anatomical and physiological specializations which make these cells especially well-equipped to provide extremely fast and precise glycinergic inhibition to its target neurons in the superior olivary complex and ventral nucleus of the lateral lemniscus. The inhibitory influence of MNTB neurons plays essentials roles in the localization of sound sources and encoding temporal features of complex sounds. The morphology, afferent and efferent connections and physiological response properties of MNTB neurons have been well-characterized in a number of laboratory rodents and some carnivores. Furthermore, the MNTB has been positively identified in all mammals examined, ranging from opossum and mice to chimpanzees. From the early 1970s through 2009, a number of studies denied the existence of the MNTB in humans and consequentially, the existence of this nucleus in the human brain has been debated for nearly 50 years. The absence of the MNTB from the human brain would negate current principles of sound localization and would require a number of novel adaptations, entirely unique to humans. However, a number of recent studies of human post-mortem tissue have provided evidence supporting the existence of the MNTB in humans.

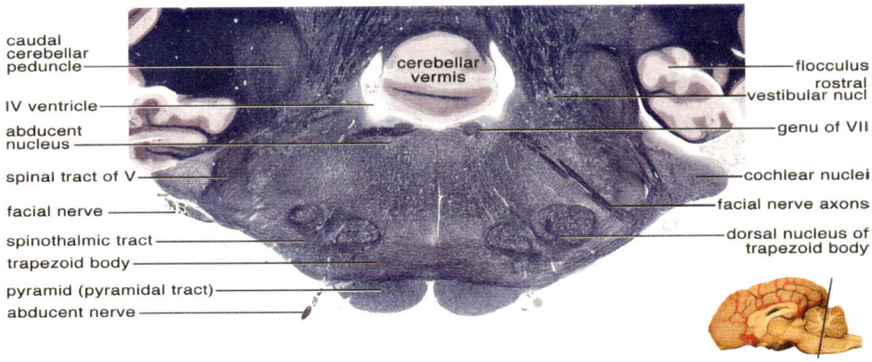

Transverse section through a canine rostral medulla oblongata at the level of the trapezoid body. From medial to lateral, three cranial nerves attach at this level: abducent, facial and vestibulocochlear. The latter joins cochlear nuclei.

Superior Olivary Complex

The superior olivary complex (SOC) is, functionally and anatomically, one of the most complex structures of the auditory system. It is composed of a number of nuclei and peri-nuclear regions that constitute an intense neuronal network with numerous ascending (to nuclei further up the auditory pathway) and descending (to the cochlear nuclei and cochlea) projections. The SOC is involved in complex analyses and filters the auditory information on the way to the cerebral cortex. It is also has an important role in elaboration of some reflexes that are key to human survival and the protection of the auditory system.

Organisation of the Superior Olivary Complex (SOC)

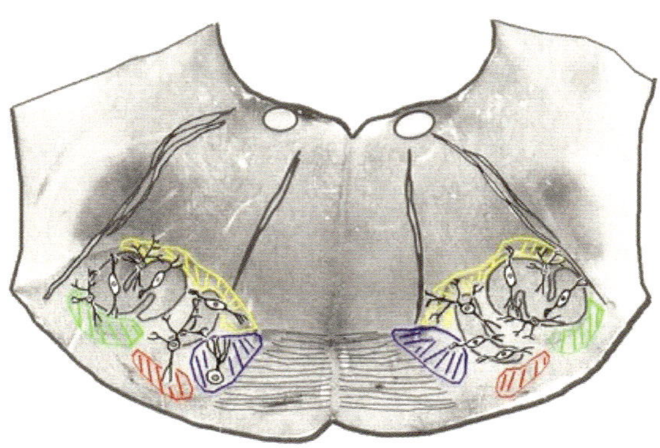

The SOC is a major center of integration and regulation of ascending and descending auditory information.

1. It receives information from the cochlear nuclei.
2. It analyses this information in its own neural circuits, even to locate the origin of a sound in space.

3. It sends this altered information to numerous neural structures.

The SOC is composed of a large number of neurons in the nuclei and peri-nuclear regions which are symmetrical on either side of the midline.

Frontal Section of the Pons (Lower Zone) at the Level of the SOC

On this real anatomical section (rat brain), the lateral olive (S-shaped), the medial olive and the striatum of the trapezoid body have been outlined.

The peripheral nuclei are indicated by colour: - in green, the lateral nucleus of the trapezoid body (LNTB), in red, the ventral nucleus of the trapezoid body (VNTB), in blue, the medial nucleus of the trapezoid body (MNTB).

The main neuron types, implicated in the functional description that follows, are also indicated in the diagram.

SOC (COS) Inputs (Afférences) and Outputs (Projections)

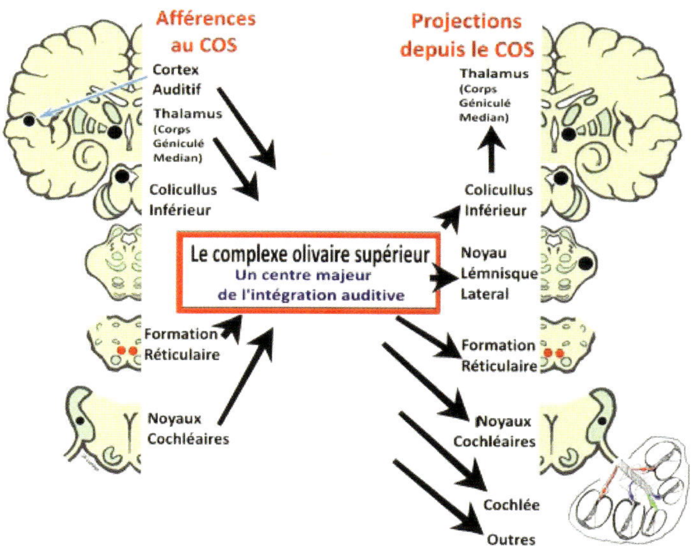

The SOC recieves auditory information from the cochlear nuclei, processes it, and passes it on to the inferior colliculus.

The activity of the SOC is controled and regulated by:

- The superior relay stations in the auditory pathway: the inferior colliculus, the lateral geniculate nucleus of the thalamus, and the auditory cortex;
- The cochlear nuclei;
- The reticular formation.

The SOC also sends projections to:

- The reticular formation to provide auditory information for reflexes, alert systems and cortical wakefulness;
- The cochlear nuclei, where it has a feedback role;
- The cochlea (the medial and lateral efferent systems);
- The nucleus of the facial (stapedial reflex) and trigeminal (tensor tympani reflex) nerves;
- The nucleus of the lateral oculomotor nerve to allow the integration of the auditory and visual signals to locate the sound source.

Protection and Modulation of Peripheral Processes

Neurons of the SOC send descending fibers (efferents) to auditory receptors and establish reflex circuits with modulative or protective roles (notably against noise trauma). These efferent neurons are themselves controlled by descending fibers from higher auditory centers.

Inner Hair Cell Modulation (Lateral Efferent System)

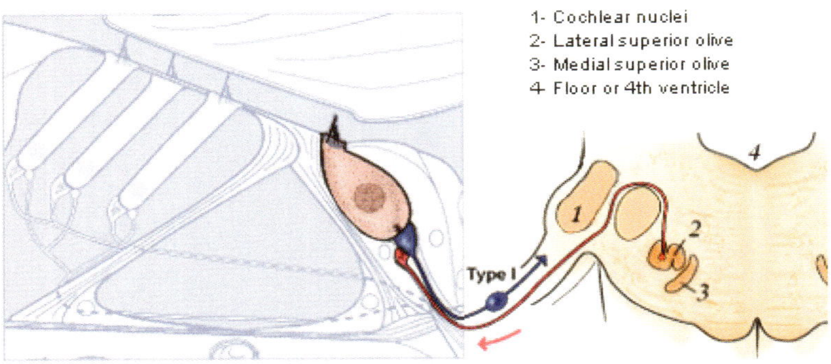

IHCs synapse with the type I spiral ganglion neurons, which form the radial afferent system (= auditory nerve, in blue) linking the cochlea with the cochlear nuclei. From here, the auditory signal is passed to the brain. The lateral efferent system (in pink), which has its origin in small neurons in the lateral superior olive (2) has a feedback role at the level of the IHC/ afferent fiber synapse.

This efferent circuit releases dopamine to protect this synapse from excitotoxicity (ischemia or trauma).

Outer Hair Cell Modulation (Medial Efferent System)

The outer hair cells (OHCs) synapse with the small dendritic nerve endings of the type II spiral ganglion neurons and make up the afferent spiral system (in green). The role of this system is currently unknown, but it may have a role in informing the nervous system about the contractile state (electromotility) of the OHCs.

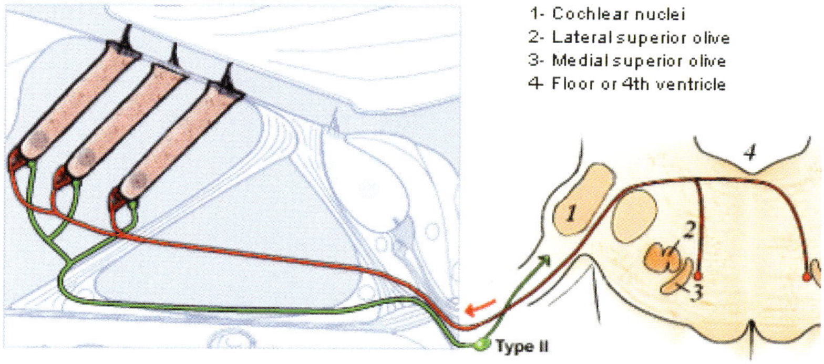

The OHCs are directly innervated by the large axon terminals (in red) of the neurons located bilaterally within the medial superior olive (MSO): this is the medial efferent system. Its role is to moderate the active electromotility of the OHCs.

Protection of the Middle Ear

If a sound is too loud, damage to the auditory receptors can occur, causing temporary or permanent hearing loss or tinnitus.

To minimise this risk, the auditory system uses protective reflex circuits.

These circuits involve the SOC and other motor nuclei in the brainstem that cause the contraction of the middle ear muscles. There are two complementary reflexes which act on the ossicular chain and can reduce the intensity of a sound (to the point of cancelling it):

- The stapedial reflex (the most important in humans) uses the facial nerve to cause the stapedial muscle to contract. It occurs for sounds louder than 80 dB.
- Contraction of the tensor tympani is the second reflex, activated via the trigeminal nerve (V cranial nerve). This reflex is activated in the case of extremely loud sounds, but is less important in humans.

Function

Upon detection of a loud sound (> 80dB), the cochlea transmits information to the brainstem nuclei (cochlear and SOC). A reflex loop activates the contraction of the middle ear muscles (in humans, however, only the stapedial muscle contracts). This leads to increased rigidity in the ossicular chain, which limits movement at low and mid-frequencies (below 2 kHz) and causes a decrease in the energy transmitted to the inner ear. This reflex does not protect against high-frequency noise damage.

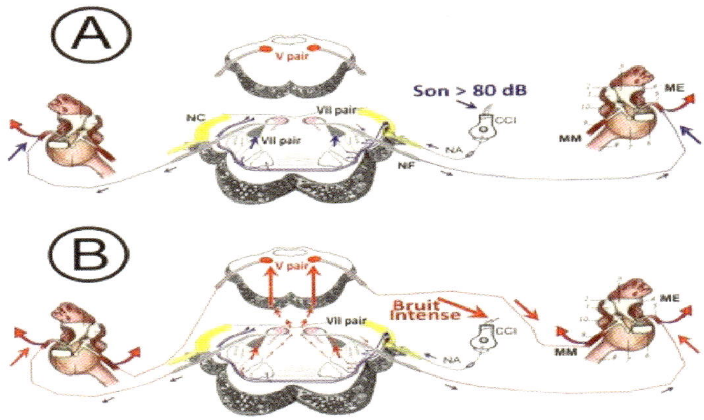

Figure: A) Stapedial reflex pathway / B) Tensor tympani reflex pathway

The middle ear reflexes decrease the transfer of information between the external ear and the cochlea; they protect the cochlea against acoustic overstimulation with the following limitations:

- They can fatigue and do not offer protection against long sounds.
- They are most useful for low frequencies, with little protection over 1kHz.
- They do not offer protection against explosive sounds (such as explosions, firearms, fog horns etc.) due to a comparatively long latency (~30 ms).

Another role of the middle ear reflexes, caused by vocalisations, is to suppress the perception of one's own voice and internal sounds. This can be particularly important for singers.

Schematic view of the middle ear cavity showing how the activity of the ossicular chain can be modulated by the tensor tympani (9) and stapedial (5) muscles

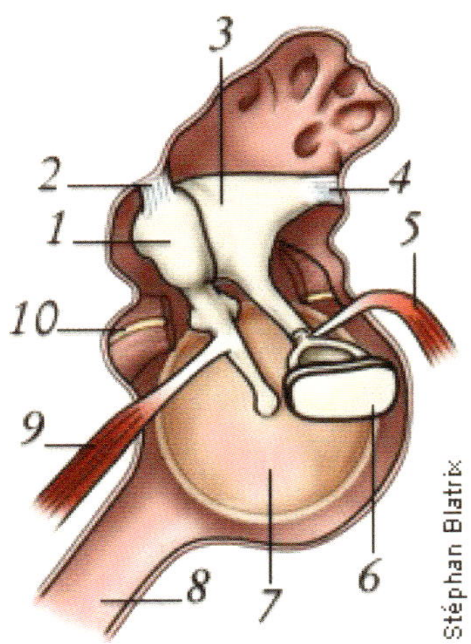

1. Malleus
2. Incus ligament
3. Incus
4. Incus ligament
5. Stapedius muscle
6. Stapedial footplate
7. Tympanic membrane
8. Eustachian tube
9. Tensor tympani muscle
10. Section of chorda tympani

Lateral Lemniscus

The cochlear nuclei and superior olivary complex project to the higher levels of the brainstem via the lateral lemniscus. Some fibers have a relay point in the nuclei of the lateral lemniscus, whereas others project directly to neurons in the inferior colliculus.

Nuclei of the Lateral Lemniscus

These nuclei are composed of different neuronal groups organised between the ascending fibers of the lateral lemniscus. They are organised into two regions:

- The ventral nucleus, composed of monaural neurons that receive information from the ipsilateral ventral cochlear nucleus and are not arranged tonotopically. This nucleus has a role in processing the duration of complex sounds, which is very important for understanding language.
- The dorsal nucleus, composed of binaural neurons that recevei information from both ears, thanks to the information exchange that happens at the commissure between the lemnisci and the olivary complex.

The Inferior Colliculus

The inferior colliculus (IC) is situated at the roof of the mesencephalon. It is composed of two parts:

- The external and dorsal cortices, are organised in neuronal layers without precise tonotopic organisation. It has been suggested that these neurons are involved in the complex analysis of auditory information (such as language) and identification of novel sounds.
- The central nucleus is composed of a large group of tonotopically-organized neurons. This nucleus receives input from the cochlear nuclei, the superior olivary complex and the lateral lemniscus. Its structure is layered (like an onion - in colour on the figure). The frequency distribution in this nucleus is very particular, as it receives low frequency information from the ipsilateral ear, and high frequency information from the contralateral ear. Amongst other things, this nucleus exchanges information with the contralateral central IC nucleus via the commissure. This nucleus is involved in frequency analysis, but also has a role in decoding interaural intensity and time differences.

IC neurons are involved in sound localisation in the horizontal and vertical plains. Their activity is mediated by the descending fibers from the cortex and the thalamus (medial geniculate body).

Inputs and Outputs to Nuclei

The table below shows that each of the nuclei have a complicated arrangement of ipsilateral and contralateral afferent inputs and outputs:

Nucleus	Input		Output	
	Contralateral	Ipsilateral	Contralateral	Ipsilateral
VNLL	Anterior and posterior ventral cochlear nuclei	Medial nucleus of the trapezoid body		Inferior Colliculus DNLL
INLL	Anterior and posterior Ventral Cochlear Nucleus	Medial nucleus of the trapezoid body		Medial Geniculate body Inferior Colliculus
DNLL	Anterior Ventral Cochlear nucleus (and Bilateral)	Medial superior Olivary Nucleus Lateral Superior Olivary Nucleus (and Bilateral)	DNLL Inferior Colliculus Mid brain reticular formation Superior Olivary Complex	Inferior Colliculus Medial Geniculate Body Mid brain reticular formation Superior Olivary Complex

Medial Geniculate Nucleus

The medial geniculate nucleus forms a small protuberance on the lower caudal surface of the thalamus between the lateral geniculate body and the pulvinar . The anterior division of the medial geniculate nucleus receives afferents from the central nucleus of the inferior colliculus and projects to the primary auditory cortex. Isofrequency contours in the anterior division are arranged so that low frequencies are represented laterally and higher frequencies are represented medially. As a result of collicular and thalamic integration, however, most cells are not reliably excited by simple tones and are probably involved in complex feature detection.

The posterior division receives input from the pericentral nucleus of the inferior colliculus and projects to the secondary auditory cortex. These projections are also tonotopically arranged. More broadly tuned and sensitive to habituation, this pathway may convey information about moving or novel stimuli that direct auditory attention.

The medial (magnocellular) division receives afferents from the external nucleus of the inferior colliculus and projects to association areas of the auditory cortex. It contains cells that are broadly tuned to auditory and other sensory stimuli, including vestibular and somesthetic inputs. The medial division projects to temporal and parietal association areas and to the amygdala, putamen, and pallidum. In view of the multisensory convergence that occurs in this pathway, it may be a part of the reticular activating system.

Auditory Cortex

Human auditory cortex represents 8% of the surface of the cerebral cortex. Unlike other cerebral areas, there are key structural differences between the auditory cortices of different mammalian species, as well as between apes and humans.

Anatomy of Human Auditory Cortex

The human auditory cortex can be studied using functional magnetic resonance imaging (fMRI), and is divided into more than a dozen different regions surrounding Heschl's gyrus in the superior part of the temporal lobe. Auditory cortex, narrower in humans than in other mammals, develops from front to back within the Sylvian fissure at the point where it joins Heschl's gyrus.

Primary auditory cortex (AI) is situated in the posterior third of the superior temporal gyrus (also known as Brodmann area 41), next to Wernicke's area (W). AI is the central region of the auditory cortex and receives direct projections from the ascending auditory pathway, particularly the ventral region of the medial geniculate body (MGB) in the thalamus.

Secondary auditory cortex (AII) is located more rostrally in the temporal lobe and contains Brodmann area 42.

Anatomical Distribution of the Auditory Cortex

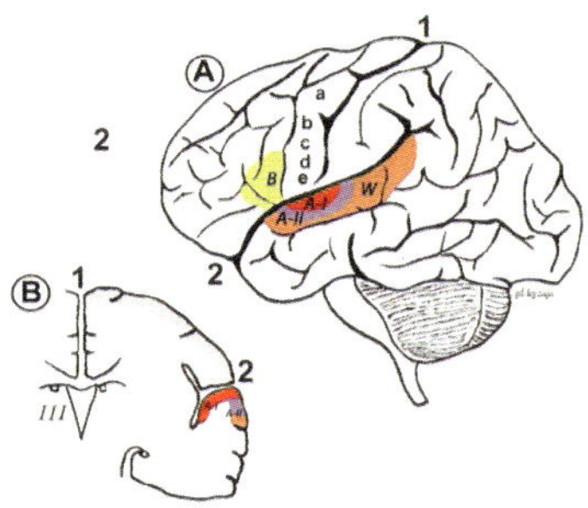

A - Lateral view showing the distribution of AI and AII and Wernicke's area (W). Auditory cortex projects to the regions of the frontal lobe involved in motor function for speech (a), the lips (b), jaw (c), tongue (d), larynx (e) and Broca's area (B).

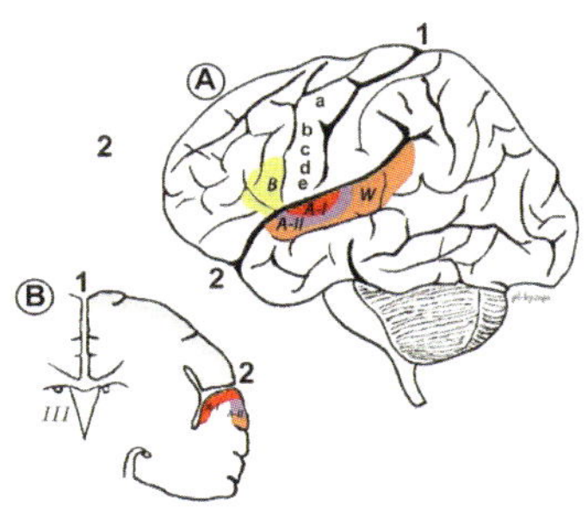

B - Frontal view showing AI inside the Sylvian fissure and Heschl's gyrus.
1 - Interhemispherical fissure. 2 - Sylvian fissure

Structure and Circuitry of the Auditory Cortex: Columnar Organisation

The presence of six cell layers in the auditory cortex is common to all mammals, but species differences take the form of the commonality of each cells within each layer. In humans, pyramidal cells (including all types) correspond to 85% of AI. The remaining 15% are multipolar or stellate cells. Inverted stellate cells also exist (Martinotti cells) as well as cells with candelabra-shaped dendritic configurations.

Most ascending fibers originate in the MGB and synapse with the pyramidal cells of layer IV, but this is not always the case. However, these contacts represent only 20% of the excitatory fibers that project to cortical neurons: the other 80% comes from other neurons in the ipsilateral cortex.

Neurons in AI and AII are functionally organized into columns, first described by Lorent de Nó. Cortical columns receive input from both MGBs and are therefore bilateral, working on the principal of summation/suppression. Summation corresponds to similar afferentation from both ears, with a contralateral dominance. Suppression is ipsilaterally dominant.

Cellular Organisation and Circuitry of the Human Auditory Cortex

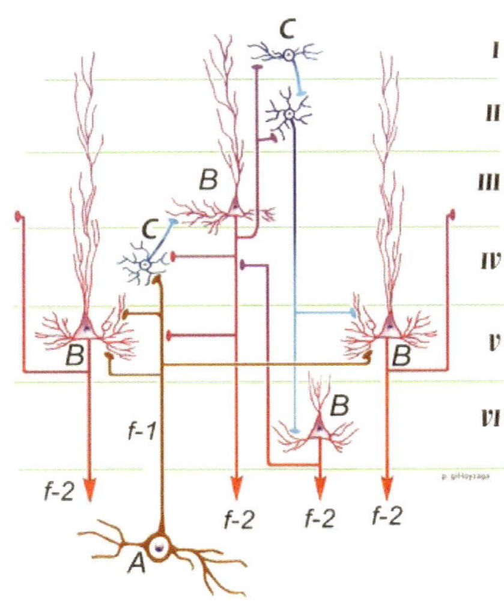

Each neuron of the MGB that projects to the auditory cortex (C) generates a fiber (f-1) that branches horizontally for a few millimeters and contacts numerous pyramidal cells (B) and puncta (C). This system allows the amplification of the auditory signal and improved analysis of its activity. Neurons in layer IV project to the pyramidal neurons of layer III, and from there the information is distributed to the other layers (I, II, IV and V) of the ipsilateral cortex and the contralateral auditory cortex via the corpus callosum. Layer I neurons project to layer II, which in turn connect with layers V and VI. Pyramidal neurons in layers V and VI have efferent axons (f-2) that project to the MGB.

Those of layer V also project to the inferior colliculus. All of these neurons also send collateral connections back up to layers III and IV.

Specificity of the Human Auditory Cortex

While other levels of the auditory pathways are very similar within species, the human neocortex is characterized by the predominence of pyramidal cells (85% of cortical neurons), and some very specific types of cells such as inverted pyramidal cells and candelabrum neurons. Another specificity is the massive interconnection of cortical neurons, which accounts for 80% of excitatory synapses in the neocortex. Only 20% are coming from the medicular genicular body.

Function of the Auditory Cortex

Classically, two main functional regions have been described in auditory cortex:

- Primary auditory cortex (AI)- composed of neurons involved in decoding the cochleotopic and tonotopic spatial representation of a stimulus.
- Secondary auditory cortex (AII)- which doesn't have clear tonotopic organisation but has an important role in sound localisation and analysis of complex sounds: in particular for specific animal vocalisations and human language- It also has a role in auditory memory.
- The belt region, surrounding AI and AII, which helps to integrate hearing with other sensory systems.

Function of Primary Auditory Cortex

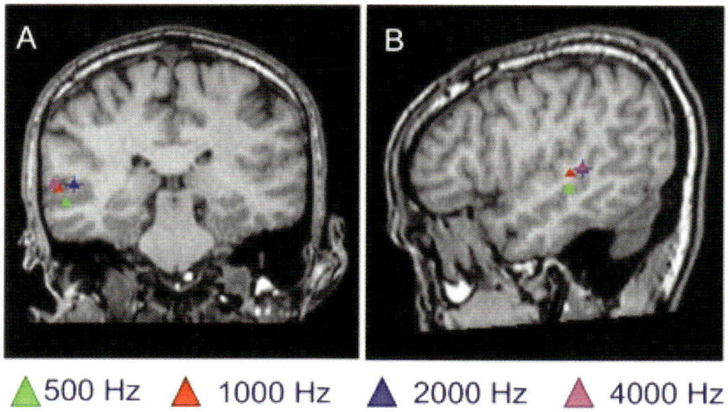

Magnetoencephalography (MEG): localisation of pure tones in a normal hearing subject
Localisation of pure tones (500 Hz, 1000 Hz, 2000 Hz and 4000 Hz) in frontal (A) and lateral (B) planes.

In AI, neurons are selective for particular frequencies and are arranged in isofrequency bands that are tonotopically organised. The precise spatial distribution of the isofrequency bands is related to the organisation of the auditory receptors. Their activity depends upon the characteristics of the stimulus: frequency, intensity and position of the sound source in space. Functionally, this region is strongly influenced by the waking state of the subject. A number of very specific neurons in AI are also involved in the analysis of complex sounds.

New techniques for studying the cerebral cortex (functional magnetic resonance imaging: fMRI; positron emission tomography: PET; and magnetoencephalography: MEG) suggest that the frequency distribution seen in animals (with traditional experimental methods) does not correspond exactly to that seen in humans, although they all have isofrequency bands, as seen using MEG below. fMRI in humans suggests that low frequencies are encoded in the superficial posterolateral regions of the sylvian fissure, whereas high frequencies are located in the deeper and anteromedial regions. It is important to note, however, that a degree of variation exists between individuals.

Temporal Integration of Auditory Stimuli

When awake, humans, like other animals, are able to perceive the small temporal variations of complex sounds. These variations are essential to the comprehension of human speech. A number of studies investigating AI have identified that in awake primates, two distinct populations of synchronous and asynchronous neurons (respectively) encode sequential stimuli differently.

- Synchronous neurons analyse slow temporal changes. They respond precisely to low-rate stimulation (A1), but are unable to maintain their activity if the number of stimuli increases. The fast changes in rate are perceived by these neurons as a continuous tone. They are involved in both frequency and intensity analysis.
- Asynchronous neurons analyse fast temporal changes (of many stimuli). They can determine short-duration variations and can accurately distinguish one stimulus from the next.

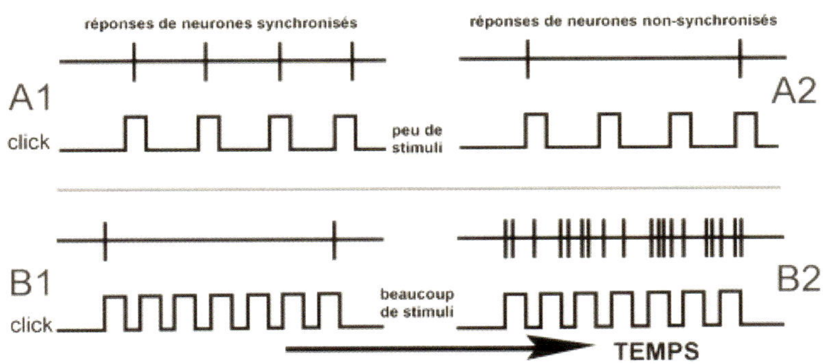

Figure: Reponses des neurones synchronises --> Responses in synchronous cells
Reponses des neurones non-synchronises --> Responses in asynchronous cells
Peu de stimuli --> few stimuli
Beaucoup de stimuli --> many stimuli
Temps --> Time

The functional division of the auditory cortex enables temporal variations of a stimulus to be decoded extremely accurately compared to other centers of the auditory pathway. It allows more information to be obtained about complex sounds, as well as the location of a sound source and its motion.

Synchronous and Asynchronous Neurons

- Synchronous neurons always respond to each stimulus (click) when the stimulus trains have intervals greater than 20 ms (A1). As the intertrain interval decreases (i.e. the repetition rate gets faster), these neurons start to desychronise their firing rate. When the interstimulus interval falls below 10 ms (B1), these neurons only fire at the beginning and the end of the stimulus (onset and offset responses, respectively).
- Asynchronous neurons do not respond synchronously to stimuli (A2 and B2), but their activity increases progressively to a very high discharge rate (B2).

Spectral Integration of Auditory Stimuli

Animal vocalisations and human language vary greatly between individuals. Voluntary and involuntary variations also exist within the same subject. Although the perception of auditory messages requires analysis of the frequencies that make up a complex sound, spectral analysis is even more important.

If the sound spectrum containing the entire soundwave profile of a complex sound (the sound envelope) is maintained, good hearing and phoneme comprehension can occur, even when certain specific frequencies are removed.

Non-invasive MEG imaging can be used to accurately determine with excellent spatial precision, the location of evoked activity that occurs in a few milliseconds. MEG is an appropriate technique to study complex auditory function, such as speech, as well as the potential functional effects of cortical damage.

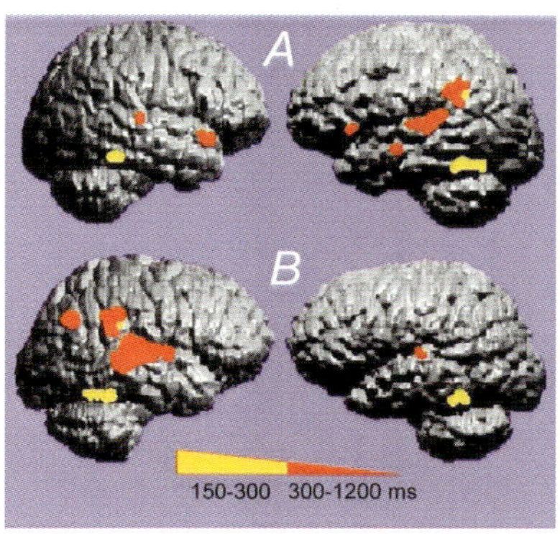

MEG in a normal subject (A) and a dyslexic subject (B) In normal-hearing subjects (A), specific linguistic cortical activation occurs mainly in the left auditory cortex. In dyslexic subjects (B), activation is more prominent in the right cortex and is more diffuse.

References

- Lumpkin, Ellen A.; Marshall, Kara L.; Nelson, Aislyn M. (2010). "The cell biology of touch". The Journal of Cell Biology. 191 (2): 237–248. doi:10.1083/jcb.201006074. PMC 2958478
- Medial-geniculate-nucleus, neuroscience: sciencedirect.com, Retrieved 31 March 2018
- Cyr, J. L.; Dumont, R. A.; Gillespie, P. G. (2002). "Myosin-1c interacts with hair-cell receptors through its calmodulin-binding IQ domains". The Journal of Neuroscience. 22 (7): 2487–95. PMID 11923413
- Anterior-cochlear-nucleus, neuroscience: sciencedirect.com, Retrieved 30 June 2018
- Stauffer, E. A.; Holt, J. R. (2007). "Sensory transduction and adaptation in inner and outer hair cells of the mouse auditory system". Journal of Neurophysiology. 98 (6): 3360–9. doi:10.1152/jn.00914.2007. PMC 2647849 . PMID 17942617
- Complexe-olivaire-superieur, brain-stem, auditory-brain: cochlea.eu, Retrieved 3 July 2018
- Housley, G D; Ashmore, J F (1992). "Ionic currents of outer hair cells isolated from the guinea-pig cochlea". The Journal of Physiology. 448 (1): 73–98. doi:10.1113/jphysiol.1992.sp019030. ISSN 1469-7793. PMC 1176188. PMID 1593487.
- Lateral-lemniscus-and-inferior-colliculus, brain-stem, auditory-brain: cochlea.eu, Retrieved 30 June 2018
- Rubel, EW.; Fritzsch, B. (2002). "Auditory system development: primary auditory neurons and their targets". Annual Review of Neuroscience. 25: 51–101. doi:10.1146/annurev.neuro.25.112701.142849. PMID 12052904
- Auditory-cortex-physiology, thalamo-cortex, auditory-brain: cochlea.eu, Retrieved 19 June 2018

3

Understanding Audiometry

Audiometry is a branch of audiology that is concerned with the measurement of the hearing acuity relative to variations in pitch, intensity or frequency. The topics elaborated in this chapter, such as temporal envelope and fine structure, auditory scene analysis, sound level meter, noise measurement, etc. will help in providing a better perspective about the basics of audiometry.

Hearing loss comes with age but can affect anyone. According to a study, at least 25 percent of people over 50 experience hearing loss, and 50 percent of people over 80 experience it. One way to test for hearing loss is through the use of audiometry.

An audiometry exam tests how well your hearing functions. It tests both the intensity and the tone of sounds, balance issues, and other issues related to the function of the inner ear. A doctor who specializes in diagnosing and treating hearing loss called an audiologist administers the test.

The unit of measure for sound intensity is the decibel (dB). A healthy human ear can hear quiet sounds such as whispers. These are about 20 dB. A loud sound such as a jet engine is between 140 and 180 dB.

The tone of a sound is measured in cycles per second. The unit of measure for tone is Hertz (Hz). Low bass tones measure around 50 Hz. Humans can hear tones between 20-20,000 Hz. Human speech generally falls in the 500-3,000 Hz range.

Subjective audiometry: Subjective audiometry requires the cooperation of the subject and relies upon subjective responses which may be both qualitative and quantitative. It includes various kinds of testing, such as: differential testing, pure tone audiometry, Threshold Equalizing Noise (TEN) tests, Masking Level Difference (MLD) tests, Psychoacoustic (or Psychophysical) Tuning Curve tests, Békésy audiometry and speech audiometry. Speech audiometry, a diagnostic hearing test designed to test word or speech recognition, has become a fundamental tool in hearing-loss assessment.

Objective audiometry: Objective audiometry is based on physical, acoustic or electrophysiologic measurements and does not depend on the cooperation or subjective responses of the subject. Examples of objective audiometry are caloric stimulation/reflex tests, electronystagmography and acoustic immittance audiometry. Immittance audiometry evaluates middle ear function by static immittance, tympanometry, and the measurement of acoustic reflex threshold sensitivity. Other examples of objective audiometry are evoked potential audiometry (CAEP audiometry, ABR and ASSR audiometry), otoacoustic emission audiometry and in situ audiometry.

Both air conduction and bone conduction of sounds are evaluated by audiometry. Air conduction establishes the extent of sound transmission through the bones of the middle ear. The results of a bone conduction test determine how soft a sound an individual can hear over several frequencies or pitches. Bone conduction audiometry determines the extent to which there is neurosensory hearing loss. An individual with a neurosensory loss may be able to hear sounds but not understand them. Since those with hearing losses often cannot hear sounds at normal decibel levels, intensities as high as 115 dB are used to assess the extent of air conduction loss and as high as 70 dB for bone conduction loss. The difference between bone conduction loss and neurosensory hearing loss is called the air-bone gap.

The most common method of assessing hearing ability is with the audiometer. Audiometric testing with the audiometer is performed while the patient sits in a soundproof booth and the examiner outside the booth communicates to the patient with a microphone. The patient wears headphones when air conduction is tested and a vibrating earpiece behind the ear next to the mastoid bone or along the forehead when bone conduction is tested. One ear is tested at a time, and a technique called masking, in which noise is presented to the ear not being tested, assures the examiner that only one ear is tested at a time. Through the headphones or earpiece pure sounds in both frequency and intensity are transmitted to the patient and the threshold at which the patient can hear for each frequency is established. The patient signals an ability to hear a sound by raising a hand or finger.

When the child is capable of understanding and responding to words, speech discrimination is also assessed as part of audiometry. Speech discrimination establishes one's ability to understand consonant sounds. In speech discrimination testing, two syllable words are read to and then repeated by the patient. This is an important part of audiometry, since much of a child's learning depends on the ability to discriminate speech. Older children of ten to 12 years of age have speech recognition comparable to adults and do well with speech discrimination testing. To insure that speech discrimination only is being assessed, this part of the hearing test is done at decibel levels of 30 to 40 decibels, higher than that of everyday conversation. By age five most children can do some type of speech discrimination testing.

Speech discrimination in the child of three to six years of age may be tested by having the child look at pictures of common objects as a monosyllabic word is read to him or her. The child indicates comprehension of the word by pointing to the corresponding object.

When evaluating infants, rather than testing of threshold levels, the examiner establishes the minimum response level at which the child responds to auditory stimuli. The minimum intensity level at which a neonate responds to sound is 25 dBs. This minimum level gradually decreases through infancy and at 36 months most children respond to sound intensities of less than 10 dBs.

For the young infant under four months of age, audiologists employ behavioral observation audiometry (BOA). The audiologist observes startle responses and motor reflex changes in the child as various noisemakers are employed to elicit these responses. The difficulty with this test is that the noises used are not standardized in frequency or intensity.

Visual reinforcement audiology (VRA) testing evaluates the hearing of infants from six months to two years. Sounds of varying intensity are presented to one of two speakers as the child sits on a parent's lap. If a sound is heard by the child, then he or she turns toward the appropriate speaker and is rewarded by a visual stimulus, such as an animated toy or a flashing light, although video images have been used for older children.

As the child gets older, condition play audiometry (CPA) is useful. The child is instructed to listen for a sound and to respond when a sound is heard by doing varying tasks, such as placing a ball in a cup or placing a peg in a pegboard, when the auditory stimulus is heard. Headphones may be worn by the child for this type of testing.

Because a reliable subjective response is difficult or impossible in a young patient electrophysiological testing is often performed. Electrophysiological testing is a reliable and nonbehavioral method to assess hearing loss in infants and young children and can be done while the child is either sleeping or under sedation. Some electrophysiological

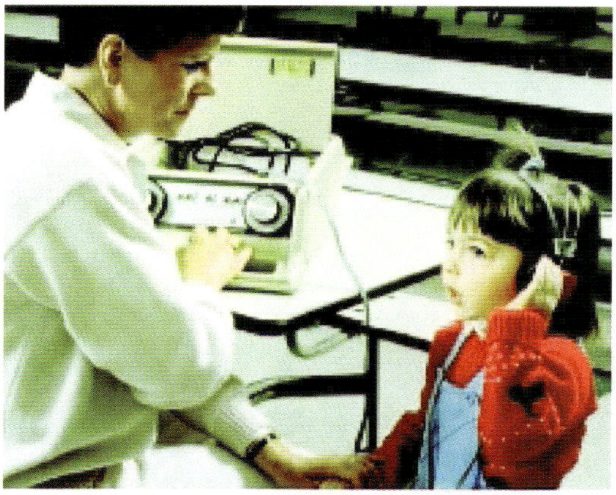

Technician testing a young girl's hearing with an audiometer.

tests are the auditory brainstem response (ABR) test, auditory steady-state response (ASSR) testing, electroencephalic audiometry (EEG) test, and otoacoustic emission testing (OAE).

To perform the auditory brainstem response (ABR) test, headphones are placed on the infant or child and electrophysiological responses from the scalp and ears are recorded in response to tones sent through the headphones. A computer compiles the findings into a waveform that gives the examiner information about the location of a hearing problem anywhere along this pathway from the ear canal to the brainstem. This test is also called the brainstem auditory evoked response.

Auditory steady-state response (ASSR) testing also involves monitoring recorded responses from the scalp of tones at varying frequencies. This test is a more sensitive test than the ABR and can also measure residual hearing better. The EEG or electroencephalic audiometry test measures tone loss but cannot locate the site of a hearing loss. Otoacoustic emission testing (OAE) records spontaneous emissions from the ear and can detect middle ear problems. It is simpler than ABR, and it can be used to screen infants for severe hearing losses, since if hearing loss of greater than 40 dBs exist, no emission will be recorded.

An adjunct test of audiometry is acoustic immitance testing which assesses the facility with which sound can travel from the external ear to the cochlea inside the ear. The most familiar of this type of testing is the tympanogram, which determines if fluid has built up behind the eardrum.

Why Audiometry is Performed

An audiometry test is performed to determine how well you can hear. This may be done as part of a routine screening or in response to a noticeable loss of hearing.

The common causes of hearing loss include:

- Birth defects;
- Chronic ear infections;
- Inherited conditions, such as otosclerosis, which occurs when an abnormal growth of bone prevents structures within the ear from functioning properly;
- An injury to the ear;
- Inner ear diseases, such as Ménière's disease or an autoimmune disease that affect the inner ear;
- Regular exposure to loud noises;
- A ruptured eardrum.

Damage to the ear or exposure to loud sounds for a long period can cause hearing loss. Sounds louder than 85 dB, such as you hear at a rock concert, can cause hearing loss after only a few hours. It's good to use hearing protection, such as foam earplugs, if you're exposed to loud music or industrial noise on a regular basis.

Sensorineural hearing loss occurs when hair cells in the cochlea aren't working properly. The cochlea is the part of the ear that translates sound vibrations into nerve impulses to be sent to the brain. Sensorineural hearing loss can also occur due to damage to the nerve that carries sound information to the brain or damage to part of the brain that processes this information. This type of hearing loss is usually permanent. It can be mild, moderate, or severe.

Precautions

Audiometry is a safe procedure to which there are rarely contraindications.

Preparation

For most audiometric testing no special preparation is required, although the first time that hearing testing is done on a child the procedure should be explained as clearly as possible. If ABR or ASSR testing is done under sedation, then the child may not eat for several hours prior to administration of the drugs.

Aftercare

Audiometric testing, except when sedation is involved, requires no special aftercare.

Risks

If the ABR is used under sedation then the side effects of sedatives must be considered. Otherwise there are no risks associated with audiometry.

Pure Tone Audiometry

When hearing loss is suspected, pure-tone audiometry may be used to evaluate hearing deficits by spot-checking certain frequencies, or to evaluate deficits more completely.[15] Pure-tone audiometry is performed with the use of an audiometer. Handheld audiometers have a sensitivity of 92 percent and a specificity of 94 percent in detecting sensorineural hearing impairment. There are several types of audiometers available, but all function similarly by allowing the tester to increase and decrease the intensity and frequency of the signal as desired.

Pure-tone audiometry is broadly defined as either screening or threshold search. Screening audiometry presents tones across the speech spectrum (500 to 4,000 Hz) at the upper limits of normal hearing (25 to 30 dB for adults, and 15 to 20 dB for children). Results are recorded as pass, indicating that the patient's hearing levels are within normal limits, or refer, indicating that hearing loss is possible and a repeat screening test or a threshold search test is recommended.

Threshold search audiometry determines the softest sound a patient can hear at each frequency 50 percent of the time. This testing requires more time and expertise than screening audiometry. The American Speech-Language-Hearing Association has a recommended procedure for pure-tone threshold search tests known as the modified Hughson-Westlake method. Testing begins with the ear in which the patient perceives to have better hearing. The tester presents a pure tone at a clearly audible level. After the patient responds to the pure-tone signal, the tester decreases intensity by 10 dB and presents the tone again. If the patient responds to this tone, a "down 10" pattern is employed, with the tester decreasing the intensity of the tone by 10 dB and presenting a tone until the patient no longer responds. The tester then increases tone intensity by 5 dB until the patient responds. This is the patient's initial ascending response.

To check for accuracy, the tester should decrease the intensity of the tone by 10 dB one more time to check for no response, then increase the intensity of the signal in 5 dB increments until the patient responds again to the signal. If the patient responds consistently (minimum two out of three responses in ascending order), the tester records the dB level at which the patient responds as the air conduction threshold. After testing the ear that is perceived to have better hearing, the tester then performs the same tests on the patient's other ear.

Testing should begin at 1,000 Hz, because this frequency is easily heard by most patients and has the greatest test-retest reliability. A common frequency sequence for pure-tone threshold search testing is to test at 1,000, 2,000, 3,000, 4,000, 8,000, 1,000 (repeat), 500, and 250 Hz.

Sound frequency (ranging from low to high pitch) is recorded on the audiogram's horizontal axis. Sound intensity is recorded on the vertical axis. Right ear thresholds are manually recorded as a red circle on the audiogram. Left ear thresholds are manually recorded as a blue X.

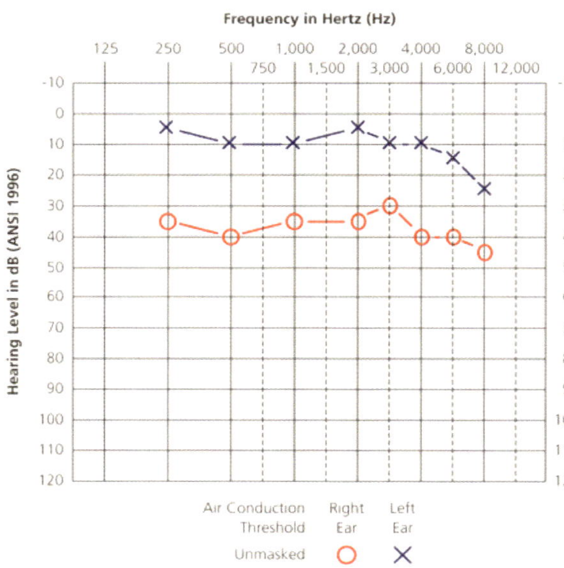

Right ear, flat conductive hearing loss across all frequencies due to complete occlusion of the ear canal with cerumen.

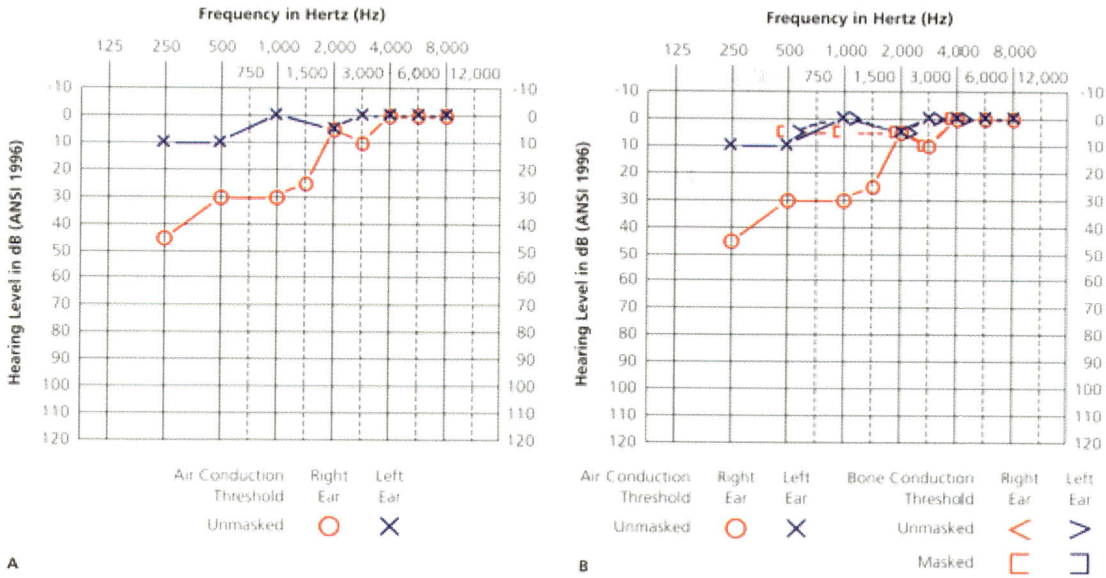

Right ear. Bone conduction is better than air conduction. The patient has low- to mid-frequency conductive hearing loss due to tympanic membrane perforation.

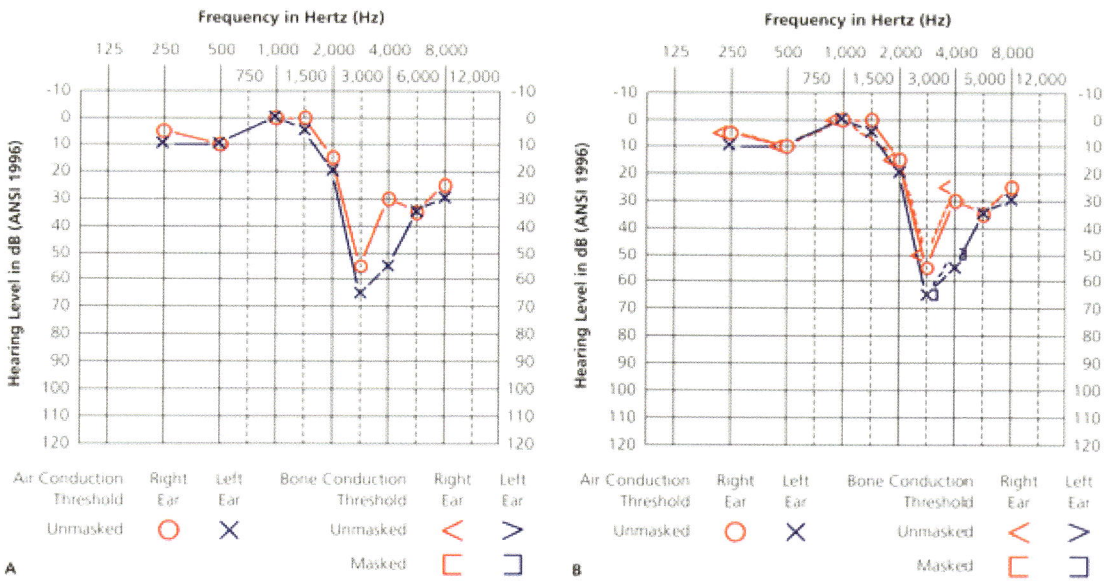

Bilateral, noise-induced sensorineural hearing loss. There are no significant differences between air and bone conduction thresholds. The asymmetry at 3,000 Hz and 4,000 Hz (with the left ear worse than the right) reflects this patient's occupation as a soldier in the infantry and being a right-handed shooter.

Conventional pure-tone testing is used for adults and older children. Audiometry is more challenging in patients younger than five years, and these patients should be referred to an audiologist with experience treating children. In many cases, the accuracy of pure-tone testing during well-child visits is overwhelmingly poor.

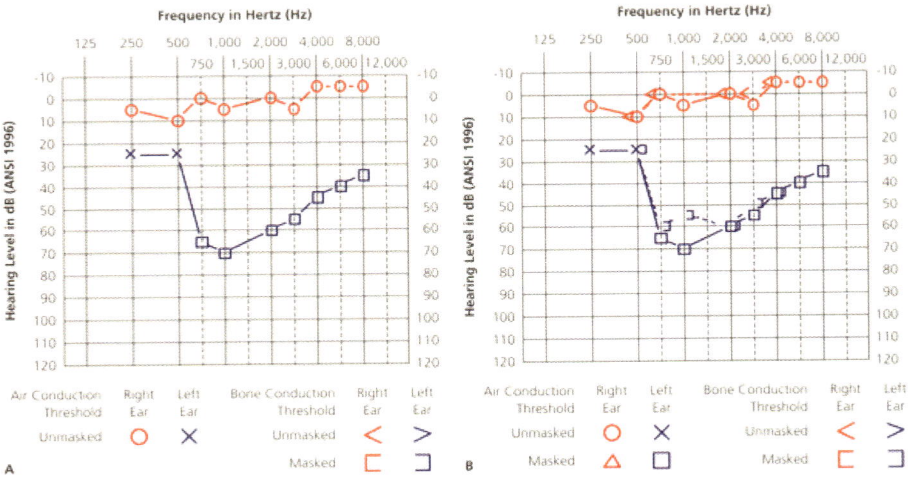

Left ear sensorineural hearing loss due to vestibular schwannoma. With sensorineural hearing loss, there is no significant difference in threshold between air and bone conduction.

Special Considerations Affecting Audiometry Interpretation

Environment

Pure-tone audiometry requires a quiet testing environment with low levels of background noise. Background noise can cause elevated thresholds, especially in low frequencies. To minimize the number of false-positive results, sound levels in the test environment should not exceed American National Standards Institute (ANSI) requirements. A quiet booth that features sound-absorptive materials such as carpeting, acoustic foam, or tiles is considered standard practice. Industrial hygienists, biomedical maintenance technicians, and audiologists can evaluate environmental noise levels in the test area using a sound level meter to ensure that ANSI specifications are met.

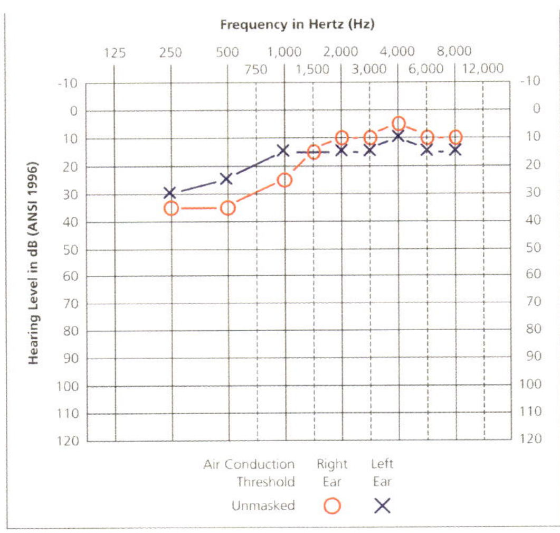

The audiogram shows a false low-frequency hearing loss in both ears because of excessive background noise in the test area.

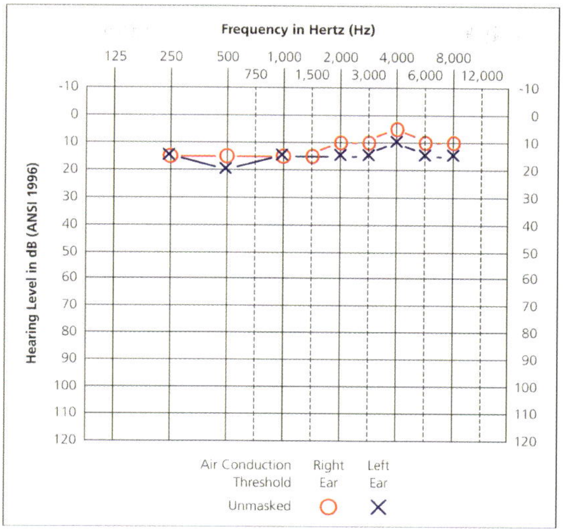

When the patient is retested in a quiet area that meets American National Standards Institute specifications, hearing levels are within normal limits.

Equipment

Several types of audiometers are available for purchase, ranging from handheld screening audiometers to those with full diagnostic capabilities extending to higher frequencies. Screening audiometers for office use, for example, generally test at frequencies in the speech range of 500 to 4,000 Hz.

There are many purchase options to consider for earphones and transducers. Circumaural headphones have a cushion covering the entire external ear. These help reduce background noise when the testing environment is not ideal. Supra-aural headphones sit directly on the pinna, and are the least effective headphone at attenuating background noise. Insert earphones are inserted directly into the ear canal. They reduce the possibility of collapsing canals, provide some background noise attenuation, and reduce the possibility of sound detection from the opposite ear.

Visual Reinforcement Audiometry

Visual reinforcement audiometry (VRA) is a test that allows an audiologist to assess hearing in infants and toddlers too young for normal tests. VRA relies on behavioral conditioning to train very young kids to respond to sounds. It is designed for children aged 6 months to around 2 to 3 years old.

When an infant has reached a developmental age of approximately 6 months, the behavioral evaluation may become the primary test in the battery. Visual reinforcement audiometry (VRA) can be used to obtain behavioral thresholds for pure-tone stimuli that approximate adult values. VRA capitalizes on a child's natural instinct to respond to auditory stimuli by turning toward the stimuli. When a child responds by turning, reinforcement is provided for that response with the momentary lighting and activation of a motorized toy. VRA is an operant-conditioned response. That is, the desired behavior is rewarded, thus increasing the likelihood that the behavior will continue. With VRA, we hope the head-turn response will continue until we have completed the audiogram.

VRA uses a machine called an audiometer to test a child's hearing threshold levels. Standard pure tone audiometers use headphones and a feedback button, so they are not practical for young kids. VRA replaces the headphones with earphones (usually with foam tips) or sound field speakers. Visual reinforcers such as video animations or lighted toys are placed 90-degrees to each side of the patient to "train" the child to look toward the direction of the sound.

Video reinforcement audiometry uses a machine called an audiometer to assess a child's hearing threshold levels. A standard pure tone audiometer uses headphones and a feedback button so a patient can respond to different sound levels. Because the device is too complex for very young children, VRA usually includes the following modifications:

- Earphones: Young children don't respond well to normal headphones, so VRA relies on transducers inserted into the child's ears. They may have either foam tips or personal ear molds made for your child's ears. Earphones may also use bone conduction vibration for improved accuracy.
- Sound field speakers: Like headphones, earphones may be uncomfortable for certain infants and toddlers. In some cases, the audiologist may rely on "surround sound" speakers to perform the tests.
- Visual reinforcers: Because very young children can't respond to sounds by clicking a button, VRA uses visual reinforcers instead. These can be video-based or made up of animated toys placed in dark Plexiglas boxes located 90-degrees to each side of the child. The boxes are lit to elicit a head turn associated with a sound source.

Visual reinforcement audiology (VRA) measures hearing sensitivity in infants and young toddlers aged 6 months to 3 years. While the child sits upright on a parent or caregiver's lap in a soundproof room, the audiologist plays a tone or some other sound to one of the child's ears. At first, the audiologist lights up the boxes in conjunction with the sound. This "trains" the child to respond by shifting her eyes or turning her head toward the sound source. Once a child understands what to do, the audiologist can "reward" the child by briefly delaying the visual stimuli.

During the test, the audiologist reduces the intensity of both the sound and the stimuli until the child's minimum hearing threshold is reached. Tests continue using different frequencies until the audiologist has a complete set of data about your child's hearing in both ears.

Conditioning the Child

There are many ways to optimize the chances of getting a complete, valid test. One of the most important is to adhere to the principles of operant conditioning. Typically in operant conditioning, there are conditioning or training trials in which the discriminative stimulus is paired with the reinforcement to shape the desired response. This means that initial conditioning or training must be done for a signal that is clearly perceptible/audible to the child. Because localization toward sounds, especially novel ones, is a natural response for most infants, conditioning often occurs rapidly.

For normally hearing infants, conditioning may consist of a couple of trials in which the toy reinforcement is provided immediately upon spontaneous head turn in the direction of signals presented slightly above threshold (e.g., 30 dB HL). For other children, particularly those with hearing loss who lack experience with sound, the head-turn behavior associated with the sound signal may need to be shaped. For children with severe hearing loss, a vibratory signal (e.g., a 250-Hz or 500-Hz bone-conducted signal at 40 or 50 dB HL) may need to be used in conjunction with the acoustic signal so that the infant will associate the test stimulus with the reward. Once the child has demonstrated understanding of the task (i.e, test stimulus head turn...reward), then stimulus levels can be decreased and threshold can be bracketed in standard audiometric fashion.

Research has shown that once conditioning is established the MRL or threshold is not influenced by type of stimulus (e.g., complex signals vs. pure tones), as it is in when behavioral responsiveness is simply observed. Infants will respond at near-threshold levels for tones, as they will for noise bands and speech. Another important finding is that VRA does not require localization skills. Once conditioned, the infant continues to look to the reinforcement, regardless of the signal source. Thus, earphone testing, especially with light-weight insert earphones, can be quite successful. It is likely, however, that localization (and its counterpart under earphones, lateralization) may provide cues that aid in the ease of conditioning and testing, so it is wise to have reinforcement available for whichever side or ear is being tested.

Effective Reinforcement

In operant conditioning, reinforcement is provided only for correct responses; that is, head turns that are time-locked to the stimulus presentations. Two conditions are required to ensure this: (1) stimulus duration should be consistent and short, and (2) the response must be unambiguous. We suggest a signal duration of 1 to 2 seconds, with a response window slightly longer than that (e.g., 4 seconds) to allow for responses to both onset and offset of the signal. Inexperienced examiners may tend to keep the signal on too long, as if its presence will eventually alert the child. Most assuredly, if one waits long enough the infant will turn during his normal wiggling-around behavior.

The best way to ensure a clear-cut response is to place the reinforcement to the baby's side, where a 90-degree head turn will be required to view the toy. If the reinforcers are placed on top of the loudspeakers in the *corners* of the test booth, the audiologist must judge a 45-degree head turn of a child whose head and body are rarely stable between signal trials.

Regarding the reward or reinforcement, there are other principles of operant conditioning to remember. One, we aim to provide *positive* reinforcement, so it is important to choose toys that are likely to please, not scare, children. The infamous monkey that bangs cymbals has ended more than one VRA session prematurely. Two, if the child's reward is to see the toys, let's put them at the child's eye level where they can be seen easily (again, *not* on top of a distant loudspeaker). Finally, several different toys, presented in random order, are likely to keep the child on task longer than a single toy.

Two Examiners Recommended

The optimal set-up for VRA involves two examiners. One examiner is at the audiometer in the control room presenting the test signals and activating the reinforcer when correct responses are observed. The other examiner is in the test booth with the parent and child, keeping the child centered and mildly distracted from the reinforcer. Usually this distraction is achieved by showing the baby a series of objects or toys that do not compete with the reinforcer (i.e., plastic rings, balls, puppets, etc. that can be manipulated quietly). A fairly large number of distracting items may be needed to keep the child's attention throughout a test session.

The role of the in-room examiner is important in achieving a valid and reliable audiogram. It takes skill and practice to keep the child in what we assume is a listening posture, so that the child wants to see the reinforcer toy more than anything else while still allowing her/his attention to be drawn away so that a head turn can be easily judged.

The examiner and the examiner's actions must not be more interesting than the reinforcer toys. The examiner should refrain from talking or smiling at the baby, except to provide praise for correct responses. A secondary role of the in-room examiner is to maintain a quiet environment and rapport with the parent, as well as to be available for quick insertion (and possibly re-insertion) of earphones. The in-room examiner's role is deemed so important that several investigators have refined procedures and equipment so that one examiner can do it all: Control the stimuli and reinforcers while located within the exam room with the child and parent.

Behavioral testing of infants and young children requires efficient use of time, because the child's latest response may well be his or her *last* response. Therefore, for example, if conditioning doesn't occur quickly, change the stimulus (e.g., increase level, switch to speech or a different frequency) or change ears. Don't waste time above threshold (e.g., quickly descend in level using a 10-dB step size rather than the traditional 5 dB). For many infants, VRA thresholds can be obtained sequentially, first one frequency and then another, as in standard audiometry.

Because thresholds for normally hearing infants tend to be 10 to 15 dB above adult values, some people prefer the term "minimal response level" to describe the results. Whatever term is used, it is especially important to note that the levels noted in the Auditory Behavior Index are not to be used as normative data for conditioned responses, such as those obtained with VRA. For example, VRA thresholds of normally hearing infants should be obtained at levels of 20 dB HL or better as young as 6 months. MRL or VRA thresholds of 30 to 40 dB HL indicate a hearing loss and will correlate with elevated ABR thresholds, abnormal tympanograms, or absent otoacoustic emissions.

Until recently, there were no formal, well-defined VRA protocols. Widen et al. developed a fairly structured VRA protocol that was used successfully for the systematic hearing assessment of more than 3000 infants who were enrolled in a national, multisite research project. This protocol may be modified for clinical use.

Temporal Envelope and Fine Structure

Speech comprehension relies on temporal cues contained in the speech envelope, and the auditory cortex has been implicated as playing a critical role in encoding this temporal information.

Cortex of posteromedial HG, the presumed core of human auditory cortex, represented the envelope of speech stimuli in the AEP and ERBP. Envelope-following in ERBP, but not in AEP, was evident in both language dominant and non-dominant hemispheres for relatively high degrees of compression where speech was not comprehensible. Compared to posteromedial HG, responses from anterolateral HG — an auditory belt field — exhibited longer latencies, lower amplitudes and little or no time locking to the speech envelope. The ability of the core auditory cortex to follow the temporal speech envelope over a wide range of speaking rates leads us to conclude that such capacity in itself is not a limiting factor for speech comprehension.

The temporal envelope of human speech reflects amplitude fluctuations ranging from about 2 Hz to 50 Hz, which correspond to phonemic and syllabic transitions critically important for comprehension . Speech recognition can be achieved when the spectral information is severely limited but temporal envelope cues are preserved . Comprehension of speech auditory chimaeras (in which the envelope of one stimulus is used to modulate the fine structure of another) is based primarily on envelope cues. Distorting the speech envelope by temporal smearing or compression impairs comprehension.

Understanding how and where speech envelope information is represented within human auditory cortex continues to be a major challenge, using magnetoencephalography (MEG), observed that degraded comprehension of time-compressed speech correlated with a decline in temporal synchrony between auditory cortical responses and the speech envelope. They placed this processing mechanism "approximately on Heschl's gyrus" and concluded that temporal locking of activity in this cortical area to the speech envelope was a prerequisite for comprehension. The modal frequency of the most compressed speech signal used by was around 14 Hz, which, in humans, is well within the limits of phase locking to the envelope of sinusoidal amplitude-modulated tones and noise. These findings support an alternative hypothesis, that the auditory cortex of Heschl's gyrus (HG) can temporally encode the speech envelope even at high modulation rates beyond speech comprehension. We tested this hypothesis by recording directly from HG, in human neurosurgical subjects, activity evoked by speech stimuli that were essentially identical to those used by. We were able to accurately localize the evoked activity within the gyrus anatomically and physiologically.

Using the intracortical recording approach, primary and primary-like auditory cortices (the auditory core) have been localized to posteromedial HG. Average evoked potentials (AEPs) recorded there have a relatively short latency and feature phase-locked responses to periodic stimuli. These properties distinguish the core from an auditory field on anterolateral HG, which exhibits AEPs having longer latency with little evidence of phase locking to the stimulus. This laterally positioned field has been interpreted as an auditory cortical belt system.

High frequency cortical activity (above ~70 Hz) has been shown to be a prominent component of auditory cortical responses in human and monkey . In this study, we employed time-frequency analysis of single-trial response waveforms to capture event-related band power (ERBP) of the electrocorticogram (ECoG) within the frequency range of 70–250 Hz. We explored the relationship between stimulus temporal envelope and cortical activity, measured as the AEP as well as ERBP, at multiple recording sites within HG of both the language-dominant and non-dominant hemispheres.

Temporal Envelope (ENV) Processing

Neurophysiological Aspects

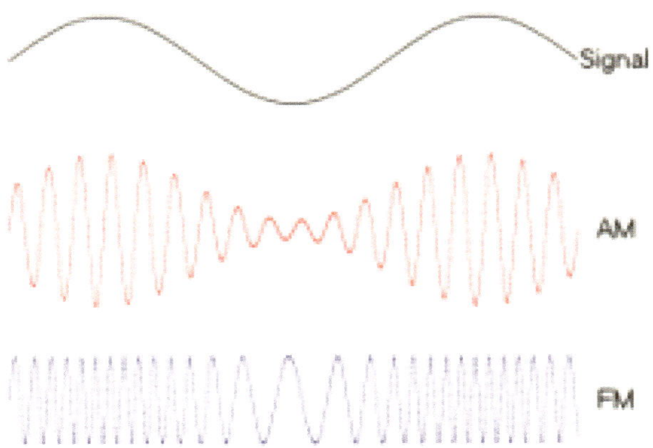

Examples of sinusoidally amplitude- and frequency-modulated signals

The neural representation of stimulus envelope, ENV_n, has typically been studied using well-controlled ENV_p modulations, that is sinusoidally amplitude-modulated (AM) sounds. Cochlear filtering limits the range of AM rates encoded in individual auditory-nerve fibers. In the auditory nerve, the strength of the neural representation of AM decreases with increasing modulation rate. At the level of the cochlear nucleus, several cell types show an enhancement of ENV_n information. Multipolar cells can show band-pass tuning to AM tones with AM rates between 50 and 1000 Hz. Some of these cells show an excellent response to the ENV_n and provide inhibitory sideband inputs to other cells in the cochlear nucleus giving a physiological correlate of comodulation masking release, a phenomenon whereby the detection of a signal in a masker is improved when the masker has correlated envelope fluctuations across frequency.

Responses to the temporal-envelope cues of speech or other complex sounds persist up the auditory pathway, eventually to the various fields of the auditory cortex in many animals. In the Primary Auditory Cortex, responses can encode AM rates by phase-locking up to about 20–30 Hz, while faster rates induce sustained and often tuned responses. A topographical representation of AM rate has been demonstrated in the primary auditory cortex of awake macaques. This representation is approximately perpendicular to the axis of the tonotopic gradient, consistent with an orthogonal organization of spectral and temporal features in the auditory cortex. Combining these temporal responses with the spectral selectivity of A1 neurons gives rise to the spectro-temporal receptive fields that often capture well cortical responses to complex modulated sounds. In secondary auditory cortical fields, responses become temporally more sluggish and spectrally broader, but are still able to phase-lock to the salient features of speech and musical sounds. Tuning to AM rates below about 64 Hz is also found in the human auditory cortex as revealed by brain-imaging techniques (fMRI) and cortical recordings in epileptic patients (electrocorticography). This is consistent with neuropsychological studies of brain-damaged patients and with the notion that the central auditory system performs some form of spectral decomposition of the ENVp of incoming sounds. The ranges over which cortical responses encode well the temporal-envelope cues of speech have been shown to be predictive of the human ability to understand speech. In the human superior temporal gyrus (STG), an anterior-posterior spatial organization of spectro-temporal modulation tuning has been found in response to speech sounds, the posterior STG being tuned for temporally fast varying speech sounds with low spectral modulations and the anterior STG being tuned for temporally slow varying speech sounds with high spectral modulations.

One unexpected aspect of phase locking in the auditory cortex has been observed in the responses elicited by complex acoustic stimuli with spectrograms that exhibit relatively slow envelopes (< 20 Hz), but that are carried by fast modulations that are as high as hundreds of Hertz. Speech and music, as well as various modulated noise stimuli have such temporal structure. For these stimuli, cortical responses phase-lock to *both* the envelope and fine-structure induced by interactions between unresolved harmonics of the sound, thus reflecting the pitch of the sound, and exceeding the typical lower limits of cortical phase-locking to the envelopes of a few 10's of Hertz. This paradoxical relation between the slow and fast cortical phase-locking to the carrier "fine structure" has been demonstrated both in the auditory and visual cortices. It has also been shown to be amply manifested in measurements of the spectro-temporal receptive fields of the primary auditory cortex giving them unexpectedly fine temporal accuracy and selectivity bordering on a 5-10 ms resolution. The underlying causes of this phenomenon have been attributed to several possible origins, including nonlinear synaptic depression and facilitation, and/or a cortical network of thalamic excitation and cortical inhibition. There are many functionally significant and perceptually relevant reasons for the coexistence of these two complementary dynamic response modes. They include the ability to accurately encode onsets and other rapid 'events' in the ENVp of complex acoustic and other sensory signals, features that are critical for the perception of consonants (speech) and percussive sounds (music), as well as the texture of complex sounds.

Psychoacoustical Aspects

The perception of ENV_p depends on which AM rates are contained in the signal. Low rates of AM, in the 1–8 Hz range, are perceived as changes in perceived intensity, that is loudness fluctuations (a percept that can also be evoked by frequency modulation, FM); at higher rates, AM is perceived as roughness, with the greatest roughness sensation occurring at around 70 Hz; at even higher rates, AM can evoke a weak pitch percept corresponding to the modulation rate. Rainstorms, crackling fire, chirping crickets or galloping horses produce "sound textures" - the collective result of many similar acoustic events - which perception is mediated by ENV_n statistics.

The auditory detection threshold for AM as a function of AM rate, referred to as the temporal modulation transfer function (TMTF), is best for AM rates in the range from 4 – 150 Hz and worsens outside that range The cutoff frequency of the TMTF gives an estimate of temporal acuity (temporal resolution) for the auditory system. This cutoff frequency corresponds to a time constant of about 1 - 3 ms for the auditory system of normal-hearing humans.

Correlated envelope fluctuations across frequency in a masker can aid detection of a pure tone signal, an effect known as comodulation masking release.

AM applied to a given carrier can perceptually interfere with the detection of a target AM imposed on the same carrier, an effect termed *modulation masking*. Modulation-masking patterns are tuned (greater masking occurs for masking and target AMs close in modulation rate), suggesting that the human auditory system is equipped with frequency-selective channels for AM. Moreover, AM applied to spectrally remote carriers can perceptually interfere with the detection of AM on a target sound, an effect termed *modulation detection interference*. The notion of modulation channels is also supported by the demonstration of selective adaptation effects in the modulation domain. These studies show that AM detection thresholds are selectively elevated above pre-exposure thresholds when the carrier frequency and the AM rate of the adaptor are similar to those of the test tone.

Human listeners are sensitive to relatively slow "second-order" AMs cues correspond to fluctuations in the strength of AM. These cues arise from the interaction of different modulation rates, previously described as "beating" in the envelope-frequency domain. Perception of second-order AM has been interpreted as resulting from nonlinear mechanisms in the auditory pathway that produce an audible distortion component at the envelope beat frequency in the internal modulation spectrum of the sounds.

Interaural time differences in the envelope provide binaural cues even at high frequencies where TFS_n cannot be used.

Models of Normal Envelope Processing

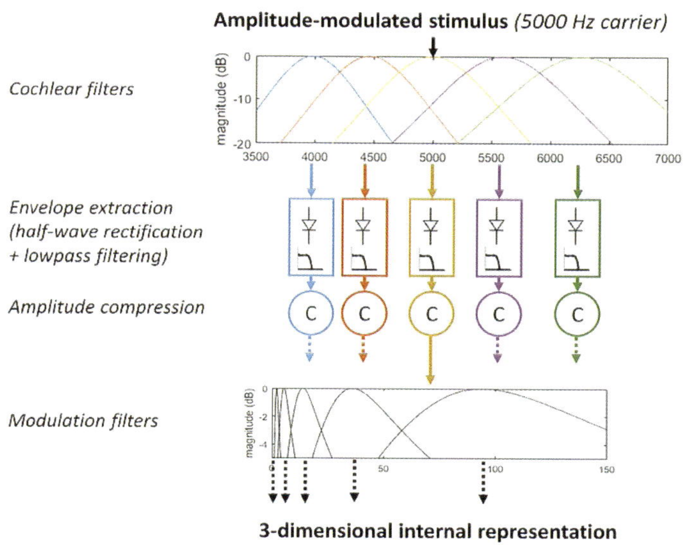

Diagram of the common part of the envelope perception model of Torsten Dau and EPSM.

The most basic computer model of ENV processing is the *leaky integrator model*. This model extracts the temporal envelope of the sound (ENV_p) via bandpass filtering, half-wave rectification (which may be followed by fast-acting amplitude compression), and lowpass filtering with a cutoff frequency between about 60 and 150 Hz. The leaky integrator is often used with a decision statistic based on either the resulting envelope power, the max/min ratio, or the crest factor. This model accounts for the loss of auditory sensitivity for AM rates higher than about 60–150 Hz for broadband noise carriers. Based on the concept of frequency selectivity for AM, the perception model of Torsten Dau incorporates broadly tuned bandpass modulation filters (with a Q value around 1) to account for data from a broad variety of psychoacoustic tasks and particularly AM detection for noise carriers with different bandwidths, taking into account their intrinsic envelope fluctuations. This model of has been extended to account for comodulation masking release. The shapes of the modulation filters have been estimated and an "envelope power spectrum model" (EPSM) based on these filters can account for AM masking patterns and AM depth discrimination. The EPSM has been extended to the prediction of speech intelligibility and to account for data from a broad variety of psychoacoustic tasks. A physiologically-based processing model simulating brainstem responses has also been developed to account for AM detection and AM masking patterns.

Temporal Fine Structure (TFS) Processing

Neurophysiological Aspects

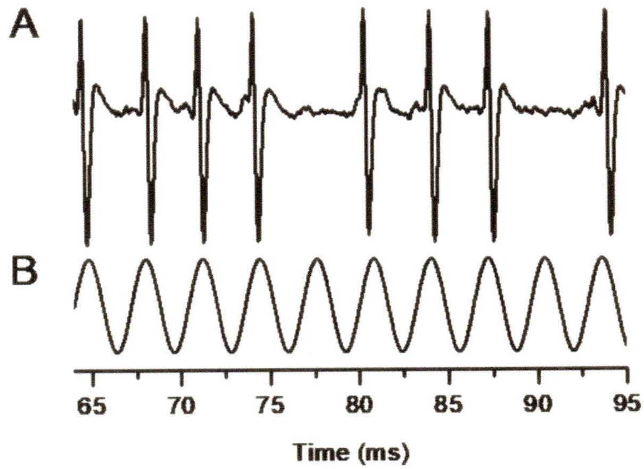

Phase locking recorded from a neuron in the cochlear nucleus in response to a sinusoidal acoustic stimulus at the cell's best frequency (in this case 240 Hz).

The neural representation of temporal fine structure, TFS_n, has been studied using stimuli with well-controlled TFS_p: pure tones, harmonic complex tones, and frequency-modulated (FM) tones.

Auditory-nerve fibres are able to represent low-frequency sounds via their phase-locked discharges (i.e., TFS_n information). The upper frequency limit for phase locking is species dependent. It is about 5 kHz in the cat, 9 kHz in the barn owl and just 4 kHz in the guinea pig. We do not know the upper limit of phase locking in humans but current, indirect, estimates suggest it is about 4–5 kHz. Phase locking is a direct consequence of the transduction process with an increase in probability of transduction channel opening occurring with a stretching of the stereocilia and decrease in channel opening occurring when pushed in the opposite direction. This has led some to suggest that phase locking is an epiphenomenon. The upper limit appears to be determined by a cascade of low pass filters at the level of the inner hair cell and auditory-nerve synapse.

TFS_n information in the auditory nerve may be used to encode the (audio) frequency of low-frequency sounds, including single tones and more complex stimuli such as frequency-modulated tones or steady-state vowels.

The auditory system goes to some length to preserve this TFS_n information with the presence of giant synapses (End bulbs of Held) in the ventral cochlear nucleus. These synapses contact bushy cells (Spherical and globular) and faithfully transmit (or enhance) the temporal information present in the auditory nerve fibers to higher structures in the brainstem. The bushy cells project to the medial superior olive and the globular cells project to the medial nucleus of the trapezoid body (MNTB). The MNTB is also characterized by giant synapses (calyces of Held) and provides precisely timed inhibition to the lateral superior olive. The medial and lateral superior olive and MNTB are involved in the encoding of interaural time and intensity differences. There is general acceptance that the temporal information is crucial in sound localization but it is still contentious as to whether the same temporal information is used to encode the frequency of complex sounds.

Several problems remain with the idea that the TFS_n is important in the representation of the frequency components of complex sounds. The first problem is that the temporal information deteriorates as it passes through successive stages of the auditory pathway (presumably due to the low pass dendritic filtering). Therefore, the second problem is that the temporal information must be extracted at an early stage of the auditory pathway. No such stage has currently been identified although there are theories about how temporal information can be converted into rate information.

Psychoacoustical Aspects

It is often assumed that many perceptual capacities rely on the ability of the monaural and binaural auditory system to encode and use TFS_n cues evoked by components in sounds with frequencies below about 1–4 kHz. These capacities include discrimination of frequency, discrimination of the fundamental frequency of harmonic sounds, detection of FM at rates below 5 Hz, melody recognition for sequences of pure tones and complex tones, lateralization and localization of pure tones and complex tones, and segregation of concurrent harmonic sounds (such as speech sounds). It appears that TFS_n cues require correct tonotopic (place) representation to be processed optimally by the auditory system. Moreover, musical pitch perception has been demonstrated for complex tones with all harmonics above 6 kHz, demonstrating that it is not entirely dependent on neural phase locking to TFS_{BM} (i.e., TFS_n) cues.

As for FM detection, the current view assumes that in the normal auditory system, FM is encoded via TFS_n cues when the FM rate is low (<5 Hz) and when the carrier frequency is below about 4 kHz, and via ENV_n cues when the FM is fast or when the carrier frequency is higher than 4 kHz. This is supported by single-unit recordings in the low brainstem. According to this view, TFS_n cues are not used to detect FM with rates above about 10 Hz because the mechanism decoding the TFS_n information is "sluggish" and cannot track rapid changes in frequency. Several studies have shown that auditory sensitivity to slow FM at low carrier frequency is associated with speech identification for both normal-hearing and hearing-impaired individuals when speech reception is limited by acoustic degradations (e.g., filtering) or concurrent speech sounds. This suggests that robust speech intelligibility is determined by accurate processing of TFS_n cues.

Models of Normal Processing: Limitations

The separation of a sound into ENV_p and TFS_p appears inspired partly by how sounds are synthesized and by the availability of a convenient way to separate an existing sound into ENV and TFS, namely the Hilbert transform. There is a risk that this view of auditory processing is dominated by these physical/technical concepts, similarly to how cochlear frequency-to-place mapping was for a long time conceptualized in terms of the Fourier transform. Physiologically, there is no indication of a separation of ENV and TFS in the auditory system for stages up to the cochlear nucleus. Only at that stage does it appear that parallel pathways, potentially enhancing ENV_n or TFS_n information (or something akin to it), may be implemented through the temporal response characteristics of different cochlear nucleus cell types. It may therefore be useful to better simulate cochlear nucleus cell types to understand the true concepts for parallel processing created at the level of the cochlear nucleus. These concepts may be related to separating ENV and TFS but are unlikely realized like the Hilbert transform.

A computational model of the peripheral auditory system may be used to simulate auditory-nerve fiber responses to complex sounds such as speech, and quantify the transmission (i.e., internal representation) of ENV_n and TFS_n cues. In two simulation studies, the mean-rate and spike-timing information was quantified at the output of such a model to characterize, respectively, the short-term rate of neural firing (ENV_n) and the level of synchronization due to phase locking (TFS_n) in response to speech sounds degraded by vocoders. The best model predictions of vocoded-speech intelligibility were found when both ENV_n and TFS_n cues were included, providing evidence that TFS_n cues are important for intelligibility when the speech ENV_p cues are degraded.

At a more fundamental level, similar computational modeling was used to demonstrate that the functional dependence of human just-noticeable-frequency-differences on pure-tone frequency were not accounted for unless temporal information was included (notably most so for mid-high frequencies, even above the nominal cutoff in physiological phase locking). However, a caveat of most TFS models is that optimal model performance with temporal information typically over-estimates human performance.

An alternative view is to assume that TFS_n information at the level of the auditory nerve is converted into rate-place (ENV_n) information at a later stage of the auditory system (e.g., the low brainstem). Several modelling studies proposed that the neural mechanisms for decoding TFS_n are based on correlation of the outputs of adjacent places.

Role in Speech and Music Perception

Role of Temporal Envelope in Speech and Music Perception

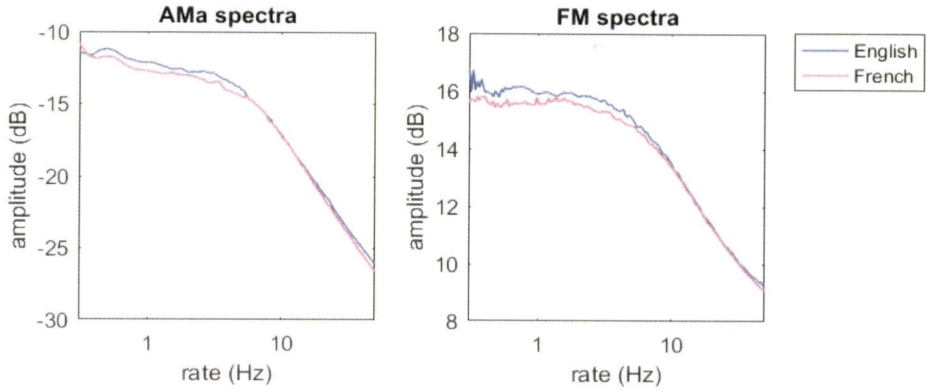

Amplitude modulation spectra (left) and frequency modulation spectra (right), calculated on a corpus of English or French sentences.

The ENV_p plays a critical role in many aspects of auditory perception, including in the perception of speech and music. Speech recognition is possible using cues related to the ENV_p, even in situations where the original spectral information and TFS_p are highly degraded. Indeed, when the spectrally local TFS_p from one sentence is combined with the ENV_p from a second sentence, only the words of the second sentence are heard. The ENV_p rates most important for speech are those below about 16 Hz, corresponding to fluctuations at the rate of syllables. On the other hand, the fundamental frequency ("pitch") contour of speech sounds is primarily conveyed via TFS_p cues, although some information on the contour can be perceived via rapid envelope fluctuations corresponding to the fundamental frequency. For music, slow ENV_p rates convey rhythm and tempo information, whereas more rapid rates convey the onset and offset properties of sound (attack and decay, respectively) that are important for timbre perception.

Role of TFS in Speech and Music Perception

The ability to accurately process TFS_p information is thought to play a role in our perception of pitch (i.e., the perceived height of sounds), an important sensation for music perception, as well as our ability to understand speech, especially in the presence of background noise.

Role of TFS in Pitch Perception

Although pitch retrieval mechanisms in the auditory system are still a matter of debate, TFS_n information may be used to retrieve the pitch of low-frequency pure tones and estimate the individual frequencies of the low-numbered (ca. 1st-8th) harmonics of a complex sound, frequencies from which the fundamental frequency of the sound can be retrieved according to, e.g., pattern-matching models of pitch perception. A role of TFS_n information in pitch perception of complex sounds containing intermediate harmonics (ca. 7th-16th) has also been suggested and may be accounted for by temporal or spectrotemporal models of pitch perception. The degraded TFS_n cues conveyed by cochlear implant devices may also be partly responsible for impaired music perception of cochlear implant recipients.

Role of TFS Cues in Speech Perception

TFS_p cues are thought to be important for the identification of speakers and for tone identification in tonal languages. In addition, several vocoder studies have suggested that TFS_p cues contribute to the intelligibility of speech in quiet and noise. Although it is difficult to isolate TFS_p from ENV_p cues, there is evidence from studies in hearing-impaired listeners that speech perception in the presence of background noise can be partly accounted for by the ability to accurately process TFS_p, although the ability to "listen in the dips" of fluctuating maskers does not seem to depend on periodic TFS_p cues.

Effects of Age and Hearing Loss on Temporal Envelope Processing

Developmental Aspects

In infancy, behavioral AM detection thresholds and forward or backward masking thresholds observed in 3-month olds are similar to those observed in adults. Electrophysiological studies conducted in 1-month-old infants using 2000 Hz AM pure tones indicate some immaturity in envelope following response (EFR). Although sleeping infants and sedated adults show the same effect of modulation rate on EFR, infants' estimates were generally poorer than adults'. This is consistent with behavioral studies conducted with school-age children showing differences in AM detection thresholds compared to adults. Children systematically show worse AM detection thresholds than adults until 10–11 years. However, the shape of the TMTF (the cutoff) is similar to adults' for younger children of 5 years. Sensory versus non-sensory factors for this long maturation are still debated, but the results generally appear to be more dependent on the task or on sound complexity for infants and children than for adults. Regarding the development of speech ENV_p processing, vocoder studies suggest that infants as young as 3 months are able to discriminate a change in consonants when the faster ENV_p information of the syllables is preserved (< 256 Hz) but less so when only the slowest ENV_p is available (< 8 Hz). Older children of 5 years show similar abilities than adults to discriminate consonant changes based on ENV_p cues (< 64 Hz).

Neurophysiological Aspects

The effects of hearing loss and age on neural coding are generally believed to be smaller for slowly varying envelope responses (i.e., ENV_n) than for rapidly varying temporal fine structure (i.e., TFS_n). Enhanced ENV_n coding following noise-induced hearing loss has been observed in peripheral auditory responses from single neurons and in central evoked responses from the auditory midbrain. The enhancement in ENV_n coding of narrowband sounds occurs across the full range of modulation frequencies encoded by single neurons. For broadband sounds, the range of modulation frequencies encoded in impaired responses is broader than normal (extending to higher frequencies), as expected from reduced frequency selectivity associated with outer-hair-cell dysfunction. The enhancement observed in neural envelope responses is consistent with enhanced auditory perception of modulations following cochlear damage, which is commonly believed to result from loss of cochlear compression that occurs with outer-hair-cell dysfunction due to age or noise overexposure. However, the influence of inner-hair-cell dysfunction (e.g., shallower response growth for mild-moderate damage and steeper growth for severe damage) can confound the effects of outer-hair-cell dysfunction on overall response growth and thus ENV_n coding. Thus, not surprisingly the relative effects of outer-hair-cell and inner-hair-cell dysfunction have been predicted with modeling to create individual differences in speech intelligibility based on the strength of envelope coding of speech relative to noise.

Psychoacoustical Aspects

For sinusoidal carriers, which have no intrinsic envelope (ENV_p) fluctuations, the TMTF is roughly flat for AM rates from 10 to 120 Hz, but increases (i.e. threshold worsens) for higher AM rates, provided that spectral sidebands are not audible. The shape of the TMTF for sinusoidal carriers is similar for young and older people with normal audiometric thresholds, but older people tend to have higher detection thresholds overall, suggesting poorer "detection efficiency" for ENV_n cues in older people. Provided that the carrier is fully audible, the ability to detect AM is usually not adversely affected by cochlear hearing loss and may sometimes be better than normal, for both noise carriers and sinusoidal carriers, perhaps because loudness recruitment (an abnormally rapid growth of loudness with increasing sound level) "magnifies" the perceived amount of AM (i.e., ENV_n cues). Consistent with this, when the AM is clearly audible, a sound with a fixed AM depth appears to fluctuate more for an impaired ear than for a normal ear. However, the ability to detect changes in AM depth can be impaired by cochlear hearing loss. Speech that is processed with noise vocoder such that mainly envelope information is delivered in multiple spectral channels was also used in investigating envelope processing in hearing impairment. Here, hearing-impaired individuals could not make use of such envelope information as well as normal-hearing individuals, even after audibility factors were taken into account. Additional experiments suggest that age negatively affects the binaural processing of ENV_p at least at low audio-frequencies.

Models of Impaired Temporal Envelope Processing

The perception model of ENV processing that incorporates selective (bandpass) AM filters accounts for many perceptual consequences of cochlear dysfunction including enhanced sensitivity to AM for sinusoidal and noise carriers, abnormal forward masking (the rate of recovery from forward masking being generally slower than normal for impaired listeners), stronger interference effects between AM and FM and enhanced temporal integration of AM. The model of Torsten Dau has been extended to account for the discrimination of complex AM patterns by hearing-impaired individuals and the effects of noise-reduction systems. The performance of the hearing-impaired individuals was best captured when the model combined the loss of peripheral amplitude compression resulting from the loss of the active mechanism in the cochlea with an increase in internal noise in the ENVn domain. Phenomenological models simulating the response of the peripheral auditory system showed that impaired AM sensitivity in individuals experiencing chronic tinnitus with clinically normal audiograms could be predicted by substantial loss of auditory-nerve fibers with low spontaneous rates and some loss of auditory-nerve fibers with high-spontaneous rates.

Effects of age and Hearing Loss on TFS Processing

Developmental Aspects

Very few studies have systematically assessed TFS processing in infants and children. Frequency-following response (FFR), thought to reflect phase-locked neural activity, appears to be adult-like in 1-month-old infants when using a pure tone (centered at 500, 1000 or 2000 Hz) modulated at 80 Hz with a 100% of modulation depth.

As for behavioral data, six-month-old infants require larger frequency transitions to detect a FM change in a 1-kHz tone compared to adults. However, 4-month-old infants are able to discriminate two different FM sweeps, and they are more sensitive to FM cues swept from 150 Hz to 550 Hz than at lower frequencies. In school-age children, performance in detecting FM change improves between 6 and 10 years and sensitivity to low modulation rate (2 Hz) is poor until 9 years.

For speech sounds, only one vocoder study has explored the ability of school age children to rely on TFSp cues to detect consonant changes, showing the same abilities for 5-years-olds than adults.

Neurophysiological Aspects

Psychophysical studies have suggested that degraded TFS processing due to age and hearing loss may underlie some suprathreshold deficits, such as speech perception; however, debate remains about the underlying neural correlates. The strength of phase locking to the temporal fine structure of signals (TFS_n) in quiet listening conditions remains normal in peripheral single-neuron responses following cochlear hearing loss. Although these data suggest that the fundamental ability of auditory-nerve fibers to follow the rapid fluctuations of sound remains intact following cochlear hearing loss, deficits in phase locking strength do emerge in background noise. This finding, which is consistent with the common observation that listeners with cochlear hearing loss have more difficulty in noisy conditions, results from reduced cochlear frequency selectivity associated with outer-hair-cell dysfunction. Although only limited effects of age and hearing loss have been observed in terms of TFS_n coding strength of narrowband sounds, more dramatic deficits have been observed in TFS_n coding quality in response to broadband sounds, which are more relevant for everyday listening. A dramatic loss of tonotopicity can occur following noise induced hearing loss, where auditory-nerve fibers that should be responding to mid frequencies (e.g., 2–4 kHz) have dominant TFS responses to lower frequencies (e.g., 700 Hz). Notably, the loss of tonotopicity generally occurs only for TFS_n coding but not for ENV_n coding, which is consistent with greater perceptual deficits in TFS processing. This tonotopic degradation is likely to have important implications for speech perception, and can account for degraded coding of vowels following noise-induced hearing loss in which most of the cochlea responds to only the first formant, eliminating the normal tonotopic representation of the second and third formants.

Psychoacoustical Aspects

Several psychophysical studies have shown that older people with normal hearing and people with sensorineural hearing loss often show impaired performance for auditory tasks that are assumed to rely on the ability of the monaural and binaural auditory system to encode and use TFS_n cues, such as: discrimination of sound frequency, discrimination of the fundamental frequency of harmonic sounds, detection of FM at rates below 5 Hz, melody recognition for sequences of pure tones and complex sounds, lateralization and localization of pure tones and complex tones, and segregation of concurrent harmonic sounds (such as speech sounds). However, it remains unclear to which extent deficits associated with hearing loss reflect poorer TFS_n processing or reduced cochlear frequency selectivity.

Models of Impaired Processing

The quality of the representation of a sound in the auditory nerve is limited by refractoriness, adaptation, saturation, and reduced synchronization (phase locking) at high frequencies, as well as by the stochastic nature of actions potentials. However, the auditory nerve contains thousands of fibers. Hence, despite these limiting factors, the properties of sounds are reasonably well represented in the *population* nerve response over a wide range of levels and audio frequencies.

The coding of temporal information in the auditory nerve can be disrupted by two main mechanisms: reduced synchrony and loss of synapses and/or auditory nerve fibers. The impact of disrupted temporal coding on human auditory perception has been explored using physiologically inspired signal-processing tools. The reduction in neural synchrony has been simulated by jittering the phases of the multiple frequency components in speech, although this has undesired effects in the spectral domain. The loss of auditory nerve fibers or synapses has been simulated by assuming (i) that each afferent fiber operates as a stochastic sampler of the sound waveform, with greater probability of firing for higher-intensity and sustained sound features than for lower-intensity or transient features, and (ii) that deafferentation can be modeled by reducing the number of samplers. However, this also has undesired effects in the spectral domain. Both jittering and stochastic undersampling degrade the representation of the TFS_n more than the representation of the ENV_n. Both jittering and stochastic undersampling impair the recognition of speech in noisy backgrounds without degrading recognition in silence, support the argument that TFS_n is important for recognizing speech in noise. Both jittering and stochastic undersampling mimic the effects of aging on speech perception.

Transmission by Hearing Aids and Cochlear Implants

Temporal Envelope Transmission

Individuals with cochlear hearing loss usually have a smaller than normal dynamic range between the level of the weakest detectable sound and the level at which sounds become uncomfortably loud. To compress the large range of sound levels encountered in everyday life into the small dynamic range of the hearing-impaired person, hearing aids apply amplitude compression, which is also called automatic gain control (AGC). The basic principle of such compression is that the amount of amplification applied to the incoming sound progressively decreases as the input level increases. Usually, the sound is split into several frequency "channels", and AGC is applied independently in each channel. As a result of compressing the level, AGC reduces the amount of envelope fluctuation in the input signal (ENV_p) by an amount that depends on the rate of fluctuation and the speed with which the amplification changes in response to changes in input sound level. AGC can also change the shape of the envelope of the signal. Cochlear implants are devices that electrically stimulate the auditory nerve, thereby creating the sensation of sound in a person who would otherwise be profoundly or totally deaf. The electrical dynamic range is very small, so cochlear implants usually incorporate AGC prior to the signal being filtered into multiple frequency channels. The channel signals are then subjected to instantaneous compression to map them into the limited dynamic range for each channel.

Cochlear implants differ than hearing aids in that the entire acoustic hearing is replaced with direct electric stimulation of the auditory nerve, achieved via an electrode array placed inside the cochlea. Hence, here, other factors than device signal processing also strongly contribute to overall hearing, such as etiology, nerve health, electrode configuration and proximity to the nerve, and overall adaptation process to an entirely new mode of hearing. Almost all information in cochlear implants is conveyed by the envelope fluctuations in the different channels. This is sufficient to give reasonable perception of speech in quiet, but not in noisy or reverberant conditions. The processing in cochlear implants is such that the TFSp is discarded in favor of fixed-rate pulse trains amplitude-modulated by the ENVp within each frequency band. Implant users are sensitive to these ENVp modulations, but performance varies across stimulation site, stimulation level, and across individuals. The TMTF shows a low-pass filter shape similar to that observed in normal-hearing listeners. Voice pitch or musical pitch information, conveyed primarily via weak periodicity cues in the ENVp, results in a pitch sensation that is not salient enough to support music perception, talker sex identification, lexical tones, or prosodic cues. Listeners with cochlear implants are susceptible to interference in the modulation domain which likely contributes to difficulties listening in noise.

Temporal Fine Structure Transmission

Hearing aids usually process sounds by filtering them into multiple frequency channels and applying AGC in each channel. Other signal processing in hearing aids, such as noise reduction, also involves filtering the input into multiple channels. The filtering into channels can affect the TFS_p of sounds depending on characteristics such as the phase response and group delay of the filters. However, such effects are usually small. Cochlear implants also filter the input signal into frequency channels. Usually, the ENV_p of the signal in each channel is transmitted to the implanted electrodes in the form an electrical pulses of fixed rate that are modulated in amplitude or duration. Information about TFS_p is discarded. This is justified by the observation that people with cochlear implants have a very limited ability to process TFS_p information, even if it is transmitted to the electrodes, perhaps because of a mismatch between the temporal information and the place in the cochlea to which it is delivered Reducing this mismatch may improve the ability to use TFS_p information and hence lead to better pitch perception. Some cochlear implant systems transmit information about TFS_p in the channels of the cochlear implants that are tuned to low audio frequencies, and this may improve the pitch perception of low-frequency sounds.

Training Effects and Plasticity of Temporal-envelope Processing

Perceptual learning resulting from training has been reported for various auditory AM detection or discrimination tasks, suggesting that the responses of central auditory neurons to ENV_p cues are plastic and that practice may modify the circuitry of ENV_n processing.

The plasticity of ENV_n processing has been demonstrated in several ways. For instance, the ability of auditory-cortex neurons to discriminate voice-onset time cues for phonemes is degraded following moderate hearing loss (20-40 dB HL) induced by acoustic trauma. Interestingly, developmental hearing loss reduces cortical responses to slow, but not fast (100 Hz) AM stimuli, in parallel with behavioral performance. As a matter of fact, a transient hearing loss (15 days) occurring during the "critical period" is sufficient to elevate AM thresholds in adult gerbils. Even non-traumatic noise exposure reduces the phase-locking ability of cortical neurons as well as the animals' behavioral capacity to discriminate between different AM sounds. Behavioral training or pairing protocols involving neuromodulators also alter the ability of cortical neurons to phase lock to AM sounds. In humans, hearing loss may result in an unbalanced representation of speech cues: ENV_n cues are enhanced at the cost of TFS_n cues (see: Effects of age and hearing loss on temporal envelope processing). Auditory training may reduce the representation of speech ENV_n cues for elderly listeners with hearing loss, who may then reach levels comparable to those observed for normal-hearing elderly listeners. Last, intensive musical training induces both behavioral effects such as higher sensitivity to pitch variations (for Mandarin linguistic pitch) and a better synchronization of brainstem responses to the fo-contour of lexical tones for musicians compared with non-musicians.

Clinical Evaluation of TFS Sensitivity

Fast and easy to administer psychophysical tests have been developped to assist clinicians in the screening of TFS-processing abilities and diagnosis of suprathreshold temporal auditory processing deficits associated with cochlear damage and ageing. These tests may also be useful for audiologists and hearing-aid manufacturers to explain and/or predict the outcome of hearing-aid fitting in terms of perceived quality, speech intelligibility or spatial hearing. These tests may eventually be used to recommend the most appropriate compression speed in hearing aids or the use of directional microphones. The need for such tests is corroborated by strong correlations between slow-FM or spectro-temporal modulation detection thresholds and aided speech intelligibility in competing backgrounds for hearing-impaired persons. Clinical tests can be divided into two groups: those assessing monaural TFS processing capacities (TFS1 test) and those assessing binaural capacities (binaural pitch, TFS-LF, TFS-AF).

TFS1: this test assesses the ability to discriminate between an harmonic complex tone and its frequency-transposed (and thus, inharmonic) version. Binaural pitch: these tests evaluate the ability to detect and discriminate binaural pitch, and melody recognition using different types of binaural pitch. TFS-LF: this test assesses the ability to discriminate low-frequency pure tones that are identical at the two ears from the same tones differing in interaural phase. TFS AF: this test assesses the highest audio frequency of a pure tone up to which a change in interaural phase can be discriminated.

Objective Measures using Envelope and TFS Cues

Signal distortion, additive noise, reverberation, and audio processing strategies such as noise suppression and dynamic-range compression can all impact speech intelligibility and speech and music quality. These changes in the perception of the signal can often be predicted by measuring the associated changes in the signal envelope and/or temporal fine structure (TFS). Objective measures of the signal changes, when combined with procedures that associate the signal changes with differences in auditory perception, give rise to auditory performance metrics for predicting speech intelligibility and speech quality.

Changes in the TFS can be estimated by passing the signals through a filterbank and computing the coherence between the system input and output in each band. Intelligibility predicted from the coherence is accurate for some forms of additive noise and nonlinear distortion, but works poorly for ideal binary mask (IBM) noise suppression. Speech and music quality for signals subjected to noise and clipping distortion have also been modeled using the coherence or using the coherence averaged across short signal segments.

Changes in the signal envelope can be measured using several different procedures. The presence of noise or reverberation will reduce the modulation depth of a signal, and multiband measurement of the envelope modulation depth of the system output is used in the speech transmission index (STI) to estimate intelligibility. While accurate for noise and reverberation applications, the STI works poorly for nonlinear processing such as dynamic-range compression. An extension to the STI estimates the change in modulation by cross-correlating the envelopes of the speech input and output signals. A related procedure, also using envelope cross-correlations, is the short-time objective intelligibility (STOI) measure, which works well for its intended application in evaluating noise suppression, but which is less accurate for nonlinear distortion. Envelope-based intelligibility metrics have also been derived using modulation filterbanks and using envelope time-frequency modulation patterns. Envelope cross-correlation is also used for estimating speech and music quality.

Envelope and TFS measurements can also be combined to form intelligibility and quality metrics. A family of metrics for speech intelligibility, speech quality, and music quality has been derived using a shared model of the auditory periphery that can represent hearing loss. Using a model of the impaired periphery leads to more accurate predictions for hearing-impaired listeners than using a normal-hearing model, and the combined envelope/TFS metric is generally more accurate than a metric that uses envelope modulation alone.

Auditory Scene Analysis

Auditory scene analysis (ASA) is the process by which the auditory system separates the individual sounds in natural-world situations, in which these sounds are usually interleaved and overlapped in time and their components interleaved and overlapped in frequency. ASA is difficult because the ear has access only to the single pressure wave that is the sum of the pressure waves coming from all the individual sound sources (such as human voices, or foot steps). To construct a separate mental description for each source, ASA must analyze the incoming signal by the use of heuristic processes. These are based on regularities in the incoming sound that result from the fact that it is really the sum of some underlying sounds. For example, the incoming sound is built up of many frequency components. If a set, A, of these frequency components begin together at exactly the same time, whereas another set, B, all begin together, but at a different time from those of A, then the components of A will be considered as parts of one sound, and those of B as parts of a different sound. This grouping is justified by a regularity in the environment, namely that all the frequency components of a single sound tend to start at the same time. Other heuristic analyses are based on different regularities in how sound is produced. The grouping of these components can determine the perceived pitch, timbre, loudness, and spatial position of the resulting sounds.

Sensation and Perception

Sounds are created by acoustic sources such as a horse galloping or a person talking. The typical source generates complex sounds, having many frequency components. [Its spectrum consists of the frequency and amplitude of every pure-tone component in it.] In a typical listening situation, different acoustic sources are active at the same time. Therefore, only the sum of their spectra will reach the listener's ear. For individual sound patterns to be recognized – such as those arriving from the human voice in a mixture – the incoming auditory information has to be partitioned, and the correct subset allocated to individual sounds, so that an accurate description may be formed for each. This process of grouping and segregating sensory data into separate mental representations, called auditory streams, has been named "auditory scene analysis" (ASA)).

The formation of auditory streams is the result of processes of sequential and simultaneous grouping. Sequential grouping connects sense data over time, whereas simultaneous grouping selects, from the data arriving at the same time, those components that are probably parts of the same sound. These two processes are not independent, but can be discussed separately for convenience.

Sequential Grouping

Sequential grouping is determined by similarities in the spectrum from one moment to the next. The streaming phenomenon provides a muchsimplified example of sequential grouping. A repeating cycle of sounds is formed by alternating two pure tones, one of high frequency (H) and one of low frequency (L), of equal duration. The cycle begins slowly – say three tones per sec– and gradually speeds up to 12 tones per sec. At the slower speeds listeners hear an up-and-down pitch pattern and a rhythm that contains all the tones. At the faster speed , they hear two streams of sound, one containing only the high sounds and a second containing only the low ones. It appears that there has been a perceptual grouping of the tones into two distinct streams . Intermediate speeds may lead to ambiguous organizations in which the listener can consciously control whether one or two streams are heard.

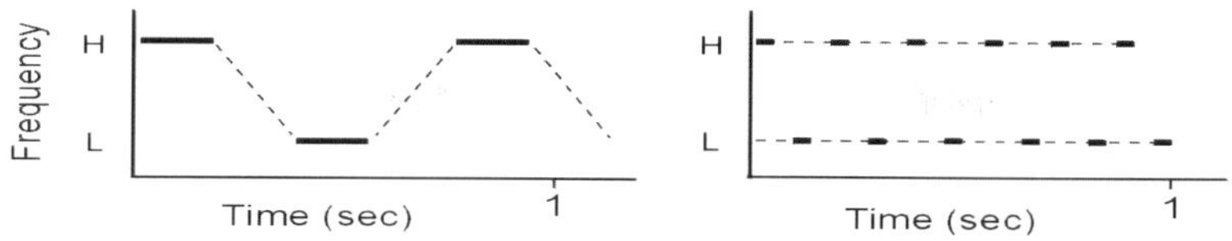

Figure: A cycle of alternating high (H) and low (L) pure tones. In Fig (i.e., Panel a), the rate is 3 tones per sec, it is 12 tones per sec. Dashed lines show the perceptual grouping.

The Gestalt psychologists described analogous phenomena in vision: sensory components near one another are perceptually grouped into clusters. The separate high and low streams in the streaming phenomenon can be understood as the auditory version of such clusters. To show why, d is defined as the "perceptual distance" between any pair of successive auditory components, A and B. It is a weighted combination of the differences between A and B on a number of acoustic dimensions, including those of frequency and time. Sounds tend to group with their nearest neighbors, as defined by d. Gestalt psychologists hypothesized that perceptual grouping was competitive. An individual element, A, might perceptually group with B when all other elements were further away, but if a new element were introduced, which was very similar to A, then A might group with it rather than with B.

Streaming can be seen as the result of competitive grouping. First one must imagine that the time and frequency axes have been stretched or compressed until a unit on each of them represents the same perceptual distance. The graphs in Fig. can be considered to be plotted on such axes. At slow speeds , the temporal separations are larger than the frequency separations. As a result, on the frequency-by-time surface, the combined separation, d, of each tone from the next one of the same frequency, two time steps away, is greater than its separation from the tone of the other frequency, only one time step away. Therefore each tone tends to group with its closest temporal neighbors, and a single sequence is perceived, containing all the tones. However, when the sequence is speeded up , this reduces the separation on the time dimension so that the d between two successive high tones, for example, is less than the d between each of these and the intervening low tone. Consequently, tones group best with their nearest neighbors in the same frequency range. This results in the formation of two streams, one high and one low.

Similar contributions to d can be made by differences in timbre, in spatial direction from the listener, and in fundamental frequency . Sequential grouping is also affected by the nature of acoustic transitions. When sound A changes its properties gradually until it becomes B, the A-B sequence is likely to be heard as a single changing sound. However, when A changes into B abruptly, B tends to be treated as a newly arriving sound, this tendency increasing with the abruptness of the change. B can then be heard as accompanying A or replacing it, depending on whether the spectral components of A remain after B begins.

There are also cumulative effects in sequential grouping. If a sequence of the type in figure is played at an intermediate speed, at which the grouping is ambiguous, the longer it is heard, the greater is the tendency to perceive separate H and L streams. It is as if the ASA system kept a record of "evidence" from the recent past, and strengthened the tendency to form a stream defined by a narrow range of acoustic properties, when newly arriving frequency components fell repeatedly within that range.

Although most existing research on ASA has been done on simplified examples of grouping in the laboratory, most ASA researchers believe that the same factors affect the perceptual organization of sounds in the natural environment.

The formation of streams has been shown to have powerful effects on perception:

- Fine judgements of timing and order are much more easily performed when they involve sounds that are part of the same perceptual stream.
- Rhythm and melody also seem to be judged using the set of tones of a single stream.
- In synthetic speech, if the fundamental of the voice changes abruptly in the middle of a syllable, a new stream is formed at the point of change. It sounds as if one talker has been replaced suddenly by another. Furthermore, it seems that any quality of a syllable that depends on information on both sides of the point of change will be lost .

Sequential integration is not only involved in the grouping of a sequence of discrete sounds as in figure, but also in the sequential integration of frequency components within a complex spectrum, for example the integration of the speech of a single voice in a mixture of voices.

Simultaneous Grouping

When sounds are mixed, then if correct recognition is to occur, the auditory system must divide up the total set of acoustic components into subsets that come from different sources. To achieve this, it uses properties of the incoming mixture that tend to be true whenever a subset of its components has come from a common source. For example, there is a broad class of sounds called "periodic", which includes the human voice, animal calls, and many musical instruments, in which all the component frequencies are integer multiples of a common fundamental. The auditory system takes advantage of this fact. If it detects, in the input, a subset of frequencies that are all multiples of a common fundamental, it strengthens its tendency to treat this subset as a single distinct sound. Furthermore, if the mixture contains two or more sets of frequencies related to different fundamentals, they tend to be segregated from one another and treated as separate sounds. This is an important cue for separation of a single voice from a mixture of voices, and is used by many computer systems for automatic speech separation .

Other cues that tend to identify components that come from the same acoustic source are:

- Synchrony of onsets and offsets of components, a cue that is useful because parts of a single sound typically start at the same time (plus or minus 15-30 ms);
- Frequency components coming from the same spatial location (the spatial cue is weak by itself, but assists other cues in segregating components);
- Different frequency components having the same pattern of amplitude fluctuation;
- Components that are close together in frequency. Cues tend to combine in their effects on grouping, as if they could vote for or against a particular grouping. Furthermore sequential and simultaneous grouping may be in competition, as when a spectral component B may either be interpreted as a continuation or reappearance of a previous sound (sequential grouping) or as a component of a concurrent sound (simultaneous grouping). This competition sometimes takes the form of the "old-plus-new heuristic": If there is a sudden increase in the complexity of the sensory input, the auditory system determines whether it can be interpreted as a new sound superimposed on an ongoing one. If done successfully, this aids in the partitioning of the total incoming sensory data.

The grouping of simultaneous components can affect many aspects of perception, including the number of sounds that are present and the pitch, timbre, loudness, location, and clarity of each. In music, it can effect the salience in perception of "vertical" relations, such as chord quality and dissonance.

There are both primitive and knowledge-based aspects of auditory scene analysis. Primitive processes, the subject of most ASA research, rely on cues provided by the acoustic structure of the sensory input. These processes are thought to be innate and are found in non-human animals They have been shown to be present in the perception of speech and of music. The primitive processes take advantage of regularities in how sounds are produced in virtually all natural environments Top-down processes, on the other hand, are those involving conscious attention, or that are based on past experience with certain classes of sounds – for example the processes employed by a listener in singling out one melody in mixture of two.

Audiometer

An audiometer is a machine used for evaluating the level of hearing, and serves to diagnose and quantify the degree of hearing loss. Audiometers are basic accessories at Ear Nose and Throat clinics, ENT departments in hospitals and in audiology clinics.

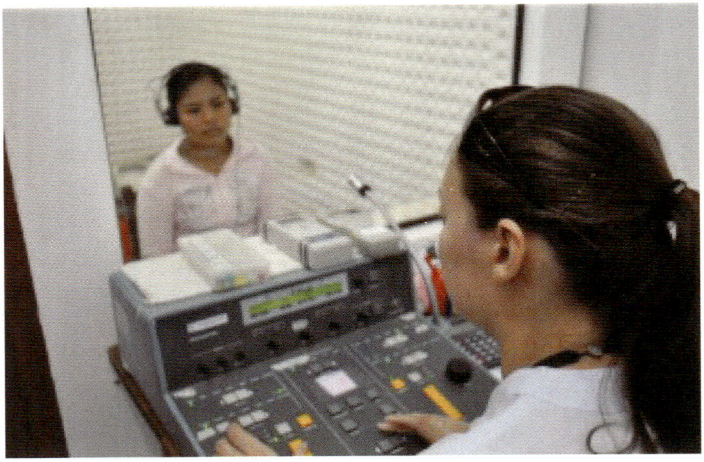

A high quality audiometer coupled with a high quality sound proof chamber are essential for diagnosing and follow up hearing tests of tinnitus, vertigo, dizziness and Meniere's disease patients.

An audiometer that produces pure tone sounds at specific volumes is used to test each ear separately. The auditory threshold for a range of tones is determined by decreasing the volume of each tone until a person can no longer hear it. Audiometric tests can identify the frequencies lost: in middle ear disease, low-frequency loss is common, whereas cochlear nerve damage is associated with high-frequency impairment.

Hardware Audiometers

Their hardware is a personal computer that receives input from the audiologist and sends output to a pair of headphones. The system includes a response button for the patient.

The computation can be integral part of the audiometer or it can come from connection to a standard PC. Sound output via bone vibrators can be applied to measure conductive hearing level.

Software Audiometers

A cheaper alternative to hardware audiometers can be found in the software audiometers.

The electronic parts of the device are available for many applications in the computation market. PC-based audiometric screening can be done by home computer and can be performed by any user of the PC in his office or home. Their accuracy of software audiometer is lower than the professional audiometry due to lack of a standard for calibration and the effect of ambient noise without usage of professional sound proof chamber.

Clinical Audiometers

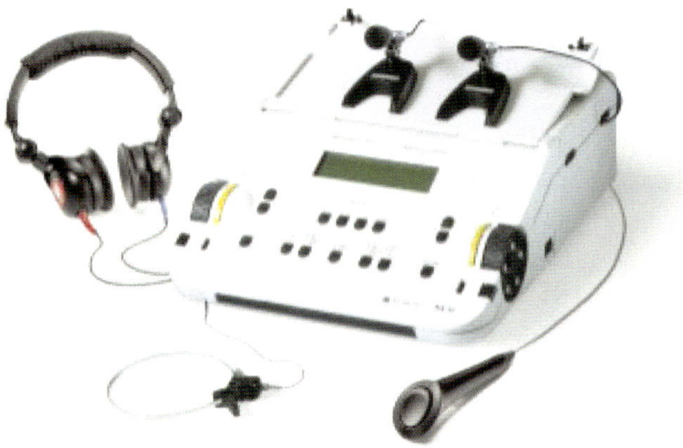

In the clinical PC-based audiometers, the higher quality of performance and the high price are part of the deal, when compared to the software audiometers.

Industrial Audiometric Testing

They are commonly used in hospitals, audiology clinics and research institutions. These audiometers perform Industrial Audiometric Testing.

These audiometers may regulate their fine tuning to an accuracy of small part of a decibel. The sound output after their fine adjustment is more accurate than in hardware audiometers.

Some audiometers are manufactured with a software developer's kit that provides researchers with the capability to create their own diagnostic tests.

Sound Level Meter

Sound-level meter is a device for measuring the intensity of noise, music, and other sounds. A typical meter consists of a microphone for picking up the sound and converting it into an electrical signal, followed by electronic circuitry for operating on this signal so that the desired characteristics can be measured. The indicating device is usually a meter calibrated to read the sound level in decibels (dB; a logarithmic unit used to measure the sound intensity). Threshold of hearing is about zero decibels for the average young listener, and threshold of pain (extremely loud sounds) is around 120 decibels, representing a power 1,000,000,000,000 (or 10^{12}) times greater than zero decibels.

The electronic circuitry can be adjusted to read the level of most frequencies in the sound being measured or the intensity of selected bands of frequencies. Because the alternating current (AC) signal received by the unit's microphone first must be converted to a direct current (DC), a time constant must be incorporated to average the signal. The constant selected depends on the purpose for which the instrument was designed or for which it is being used.

A typical sound-level meter can be switched between a scale that reads sound intensities uniformly for most frequencies—called unweighted—and a scale that introduces a frequency-dependent weighting factor, thus yielding a response more nearly like that of the human ear. A-frequency-weighting is the most commonly used standard, but B-, C-, D-, and Z-frequency-weightings also exist. The A-frequency-weighting scale is useful in describing how complex noises affect people. Thus, the scale is recognized internationally for measurements relating to prevention of deafness from excessive noise in work environments.

In the early 1970s, as concern about noise pollution increased, accurate, versatile, portable noise-measuring instruments were developed. Sound level is not a measure of loudness, as loudness is a subjective factor and depends on the characteristics of the ear of the listener. In an attempt to overcome this problem, scales have been developed to correlate loudness with objective measurements of sound. The Fletcher–Munson curve, for example, shows the relationship between loudness in decibels and subjectively judged loudness.

How loud a sound seems to be depends on who's listening. A young person playing rock up in their bedroom might not think their music is loud, but their parents in the room down below might have other ideas. In other words, how loud things seem is a subjective thing and not something we can easily measure. However, what makes one sound seem louder than another is the amount of energy that the source of the sound is pumping towards the listener in the form of pressure variations in the air. That's the intensity of the sound and it's an objective thing—something we can easily measure and agree on.

Meters that measure sound levels work by calculating the pressure of the sound waves traveling through the air from a source of noise. That's why you'll sometimes see them referred to as sound pressure level (SPL) meters. Devices like this give a measurement of sound intensity in units called decibels, a scale first devised by telephone pioneer Alexander Graham Bell.

Classification

Types

The IEC 61672-1 specifies "three kinds of sound measuring instruments". They are the "conventional" sound level meter, the integrating-averaging sound level meter, and the integrating sound level meter.

The standard sound level meter can be called an *exponentially averaging sound level meter* as the AC signal from the microphone is converted to DC by a root-mean-square (RMS) circuit and thus it must have a time constant of integration; today referred to as the time-weighting. Three of these time-weightings have been internationally standardized, 'S' (1 s) originally called Slow, 'F' (125 ms) originally called Fast and 'I' (35 ms) originally called Impulse. Their names were changed in the 1980s to be the same in any language. I-time-weighting is no longer in the body of the standard because it has little real correlation with the impulsive character of noise events.

The output of the RMS circuit is linear in voltage and is passed through a logarithmic circuit to give a readout linear in decibels (dB). This is 20 times the base 10 logarithm of the ratio of a given root-mean-square sound pressure to the reference sound pressure. Root-mean-square sound pressure being obtained with a standard frequency weighting and standard time weighting. The reference pressure is set by International agreement to be 20 micropascals for airborne sound. It follows that the decibel is, in a sense, not a unit, it is simply a dimensionless ratio; in this case the ratio of two pressures.

An exponentially averaging sound level meter, which gives a snapshot of the current noise level, is of limited use for hearing damage risk measurements; an integrating or integrating-averaging meter is usually mandated. An integrating meter simply integrates—or in other words 'sums'—the frequency-weighted noise to give sound exposure and the metric used is pressure squared times time, often $Pa^2 \cdot s$, but $Pa^2 \cdot h$ is also used. However, because the unit of sound was historically described in decibels, the exposure is most often described in terms of sound exposure level (SEL), the logarithmic conversion of sound exposure into decibels.

Personal Noise Dosimeter

A common variant of the sound level meter is a noise dosemeter (dosimeter in American English). However, this is now formally known as a personal sound exposure meter (PSEM) and has its own International standard IEC 61252:1993.

A noise dosimeter (American) or noise dosemeter (British) is a specialized sound level meter intended specifically to measure the noise exposure of a person integrated over a period of time; usually to comply with Health and Safety regulations such as the Occupational Safety and Health (OSHA) 29 CFR 1910.95 Occupational Noise Exposure Standard or EU Directive 2003/10/EC.

This is normally intended to be a body-worn instrument and thus has a relaxed technical requirement, as a body-worn instrument—because of the presence of the body—has a poorer overall acoustic performance. A PSEM gives a read-out based on sound exposure, usually $Pa^2 \cdot h$, and the older 'classic' dosimeters giving the metric of 'percentage dose' are no longer used in most countries. The problem with "%dose" is that it relates to the political situation and thus any device can become obsolete if the "100%" value is changed by local laws.

Traditionally, noise dosemeters were relatively large devices with a microphone mounted near the ear and having a cable going to the instrument body, itself usually belt worn. These devices had several issues, mainly the reliability of the cable and the disturbance to the user's normal work mode, caused by the presence of the cable. In 1997 following a UK research grant an EU patent was issued for the first of a range of devices that were so small that they resembled a radiation badge and no cable was needed as the whole unit could be fitted near the ear. Today these devices measure not only simple noise dose, but some even have four separate dosemeters, each with many of the functions of a full-sized sound level meter, including in the latest models full octave band analysis.

Classes

IEC standards divide sound level meters into two "classes". Sound level meters of the two classes have the same functionality, but different tolerances for error. Class 1 instruments have a wider frequency range and a tighter tolerance than a lower cost, Class 2 unit. This applies to both the sound level meter itself as well as the associated calibrator. Most national standards permit the use of "at least a Class 2 instrument". For many measurements, it is not necessary to use a Class 1 unit; these are best employed for research and law enforcement.

Similarly, the American National Standards Institute (ANSI) specifies sound level meters as three different Types 0, 1 and 2. These are described, as follows, in the Occupational Safety and Health OSHA Technical Manual TED01-00-015, Chapter 5, OSHA Noise and Hearing Conservation, Appendix III:A, "These ANSI standards set performance and accuracy tolerances according to three levels of precision: Types 0, 1, and 2. Type 0 is used in laboratories, Type 1 is used for precision measurements in the field, and Type 2 is used for general-purpose measurements. For compliance purposes, readings with an ANSI Type 2 sound level meter and dosimeter are considered to have an accuracy of ±2 dBA, while a Type 1 instrument has an accuracy of ±1 dBA. A Type 2 meter is the minimum requirement by OSHA for noise measurements and is usually sufficient for general purpose noise surveys. The Type 1 meter is preferred for the design of cost-effective noise controls. For unusual measurement situations, refer to the manufacturer's instructions and appropriate ANSI standards for guidance in interpreting instrument accuracy."

Measurements

Labels used to describe sound and noise level values are defined in the IEC Standard 61672-1:2013

Level

For labels, the first letter is always an L. This simply stands for Level, as in the sound pressure level measured through a microphone or the electronic signal level measured at the output from an audio component, such as a mixing desk.

Frequency Weighting

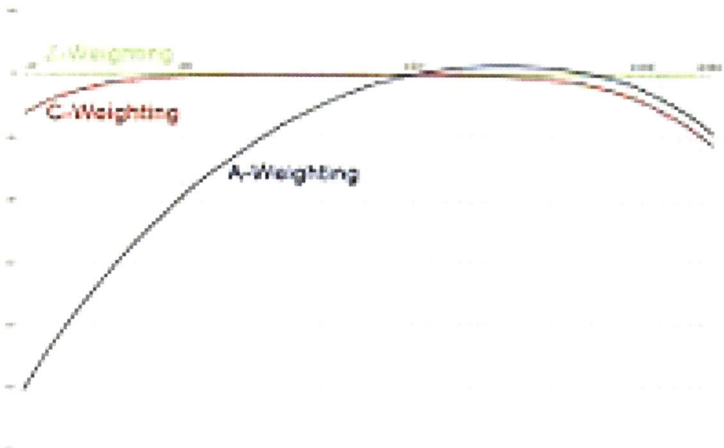

A, C and Z frequency weightings for sound

The second letter indicates the frequency weighting. 'Pattern Approved' sound level meters offer noise measurements with A, C and Z frequency weighting.

Z-Weighting represents the actual sound produced. A-Weighting, with less lower and higher frequencies, and a slight boost in the mid-range, represents what humans are capable of hearing. C-Weighting, more sensitive to the lower frequencies, represents what humans hear when the sound is loud (over 100 dB).

The IEC 61672-1:2013 mandates the inclusion of an *A*-frequency-weighting filter in all sound level meters, and also describes *C* and *Z* (zero) frequency weightings. The older *B* and *D* frequency weightings are now obsolete and are no longer described in the standard.

In almost all countries, the use of A-frequency-weighting is mandated to be used for the protection of workers against noise-induced hearing loss. The A-frequency curve was based on the historical equal-loudness contours and while arguably A-frequency-weighting is no longer the ideal frequency weighting on purely scientific grounds, it is nonetheless the legally required standard for almost all such measurements and has the huge practical advantage that old data can be compared with new measurements. It is for these reasons that A-frequency-weighting is the only weighting mandated by the international standard, the frequency weightings 'C' and 'Z' being optional fitments.

Originally, the A-frequency-weighting was only meant for quiet sounds in the region of 40 dB sound pressure level (SPL), but is now mandated for all levels. C-frequency weighting is however still used in the measurement of the peak value of a noise in some legislation, but B-frequency weighting – a halfway house between 'A' and 'C' has almost no practical use. D-frequency-weighting was designed for use in measuring aircraft noise when non-bypass jets were being measured and after the demise of Concord, these are all military types. For all civil aircraft noise measurements, A-frequency-weighting is used as is mandated by the ISO and ICAO standards.

Time Weighting

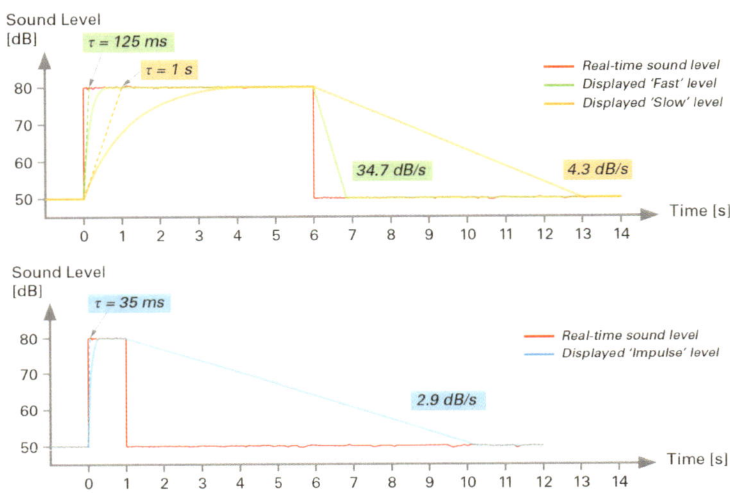

Graphs of Fast, Slow and Impulse time weightings applied so that sound levels measured are easier to read on a sound level meter.

If the third letter is F, S or I, this represents the time weighting. F = Fast, S = Slow, I = Impulse. Time weighting is applied so that levels measured are easier to read on a sound level meter. The time weighting dampens sudden changes in levels, thus creating a smoother display.

The graph indicates how this works. In this example, the input signal suddenly increases from 50 dB to 80 dB, stays there for 6 seconds, then disappears just as suddenly.

A Slow measurement (yellow line) will take approximately 5 seconds (attack time) to reach 80 dB and around 6 seconds (decay time) to drop back down to 50 dB. S is appropriate when measuring a signal that fluctuates a lot.

A Fast measurement (green line) is quicker to react. It will take approximately 0.6 seconds to reach 80 dB and just under 1 second to drop back down to 50 dB. F may be more suitable where the signal is less impulsive.

The decision to use Fast or Slow is often reached by what is prescribed in a standard or a law.

An Impulse measurement (blue line) will take approximately 0.3 seconds to reach 80 dB and over 9 seconds to drop back down to 50 dB. The impulse response, I can be used in situations where there are sharp impulsive noises, such as when measuring fireworks or gunshots.

L_{AT} or L_{eq}: Equivalent Continuous Sound Level

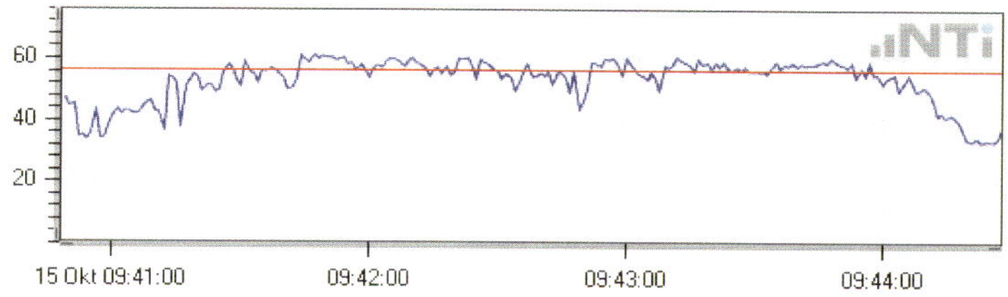

Graph of LA_{eq} sound level measurement calculated over 5 minutes

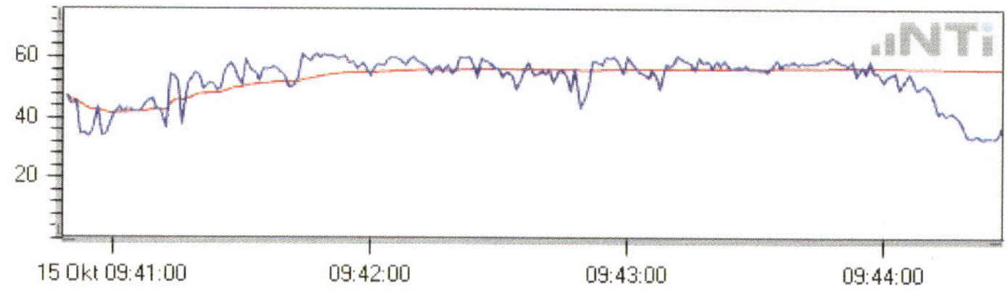

Graph of a continuous LA_{eq} sound level measurement

eq = equivalent. Equivalent values are a form of time weighting that is easier to read on a display than the instantaneous sound level.

If you look at these graphs of sound level over time, the area under the blue curve represents the energy. The horizontal red line drawn to represent the same area under the blue curve, gives us the LA_{eq}. That is the equivalent value or average of the energy over the entire graph.

LA_{eq} is not always a straight line. If the LA_{eq} is plotted as the equivalent from the beginning of the graph to each of the measurement points, the plot is shown in the second graph.

Sound exposure level—in decibels—is not much used in industrial noise measurement. Instead, the time-averaged value is used. This is the time average sound level or as it is usually called the 'equivalent continuous sound level' has the formal symbol L_{AT} as described in paragraph 3,9 "Definitions" of IEC 61672-1 where many correct formal symbols and their common abbreviations are given. These mainly follow the formal ISO acoustic definitions. However, for mainly historical reasons, L_{AT} is commonly referred to as L_{eq}.

Formally, L_{AT} is 10 times the base 10 logarithm of the ratio of a root-mean-square A-weighted sound pressure during a stated time interval to the reference sound pressure and there is no time constant involved. To measure L_{AT} an integrating-averaging meter is needed; this in concept takes the sound exposure, divides it by time and then takes the logarithm of the result.

Short Leq

An important variant of overall L_{AT} is "short L_{eq}" where very short L_{eq} values are taken in succession, say at 1/8 second intervals, each being stored in a digital memory. These data elements can either be transmitted to another unit or be recovered from the memory and re-constituted into almost any conventional metric long after the data has been acquired. This can be done using either dedicated programs or standard spreadsheets. Short L_{eq} has the advantage that as regulations change, old data can be re-processed to check if a new regulation is met. It also permits data to be converted from one metric to another in some cases. Today almost all fixed airport noise monitoring systems, which are in concept just complex sound level meters, use short L_{eq} as their metric, as a steady stream of the digital one second L_{eq} values can be transmitted via telephone lines or the Internet to a central display and processing unit. Short L_{eq} is a feature of most commercial integrating sound level meters—although some manufacturers give it many different names.

Short L_{eq} is a very valuable method for acoustic data storage; initially, a concept of the French Government's Laboratoire National d'Essais (ref 1), it has now become the most common method of storing and displaying a true time history of the noise in professional commercial sound level meters. The alternative method, which is to generate a time history by storing and displaying samples of the exponential sound level, displays too many artifacts of the sound level meter to be as valuable and such sampled data cannot be readily combined to form an overall set of data.

Until 2003 there were separate standards for exponential and linear integrating sound level meters, (IEC 60651 and IEC 60804—both now withdrawn), but since then the combined standard IEC 61672 has described both types of meter. For short L_{eq} to be valuable the manufacturer must ensure that each separate L_{eq} element fully complies with IEC 61672.

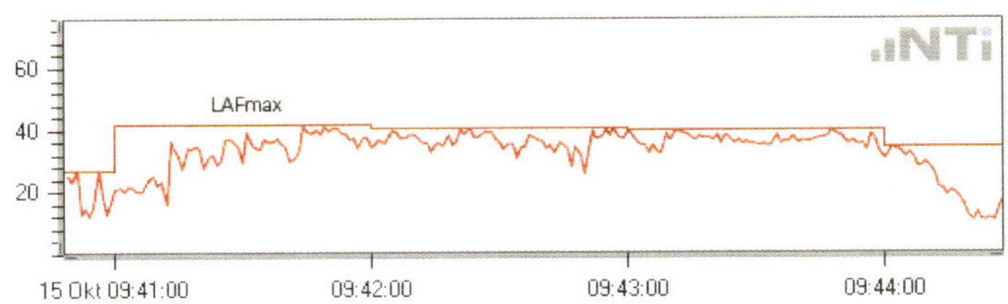

Graph of an LAFmax sound level measurement calculated every minute

L_{max} and L_{min}

If the words max or min appear in the label, this simply represents the maximum or minimum value measured over a certain period of time.

LC_{pk}: Peak Sound Pressure Level

Most national regulations also call for the absolute peak value to be measured to protect workers hearing against sudden large pressure peaks, using either 'C' or 'Z' frequency weighting. 'Peak sound pressure level' should not be confused with 'MAX sound pressure level'. 'Max sound pressure level' is simply the highest RMS reading a conventional sound level meter gives over a stated period for a given time-weighting (S, F, or I) and can be many decibels less than the peak value. In the European Union, the maximum permitted value of the peak sound level is 140 dB(C) and this equates to 200 Pa pressure. The symbol for the *A*-frequency and *S*-time weighted maximum sound level is LAS_{max}. For the *C*-frequency weighted peak it is LC_{pk} or $L_{C,peak}$.

Other Applications

Noise Monitoring Stations

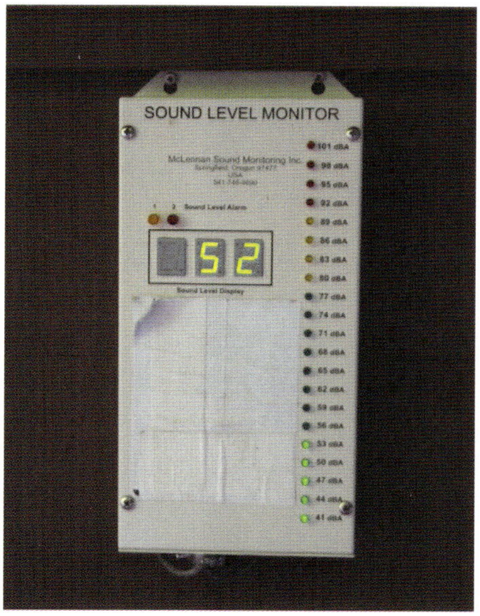

Noise monitoring station at Muir Woods National Monument in California

Some applications require the ability to monitor noise continuously on a permanent or semi-permanent basis. Some manufacturers offer permanent and semi-permanent noise monitoring stations for this purpose. Such monitoring stations are typically based on a sound level meter at the heart and some added capabilities such as remote communication, GPS, and weather stations. These can often also be powered using solar power. Applications for such monitoring stations include airport noise, construction noise, mining noise, traffic noise, rail noise, community noise, wind farm noise, industrial noise, etc.

Modern monitoring stations can also offer remote communication capabilities using cellular modems, WiFi networks or direct LAN wires. Such devices allow for real-time alerts and notifications via email and text messages upon exceeding a certain dB level.

Systems can also remotely email reports on a daily, weekly or monthly basis. Real-time data publication is often also desired, which can be achieved by pushing data to a website.

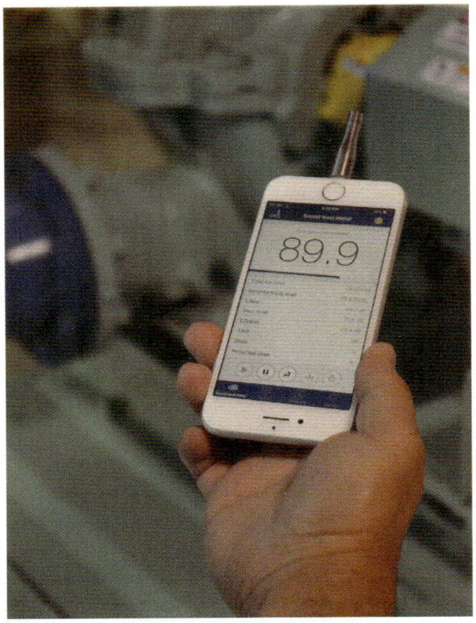

NIOSH sound level meter application (app)

Smartphone Applications

The ubiquity of smartphones, their constant network connectivity, the built-in geographic information system functionality and user-interactivity features present a great opportunity to revolutionize the way we look at noise, its measurement, and its effects on hearing and overall health. The ability to acquire and display real-time noise exposure data raises people's awareness about their work (and off-work) environment and allows them to make informed decisions about hearing hazards and overall well-being. NIOSH conducted a pilot study to select and characterize the functionality and accuracy of smartphone sound measurement applications (apps) as an initial step in a broader effort to determine whether these apps can be relied on to conduct participatory noise monitoring studies in the workplace. Although most smartphone sound measurement apps are not accurate enough to be used for legally required measurements, the NIOSH Sound Level Meter app met the requirements of IEC 61672/ANSI S1.4 Sound Level Meter Standards (Electroacoustics - Sound Level Meters - Part 3: Periodic Tests).

Building Acoustics, Sound Insulation and Reverberation Time

Some advanced sound level meters can also include reverberation time (RT60) measurement capabilities. Measurements can be done using the Integrated Impulse Response or Interrupted Noise Methods. Such sound level meters should comply with latest ISO 3382-2 and ASTM E2235-04 measurement standards. Also required for measuring the acoustics in buildings is a signal generator that provides pink or white noise through an amplifier and omnidirectional speakers. Such measurements are also used for calculation of wall/partition sound insulation.

How to use Sound Level Meter

This topic describes how to use physically the instrument in order to correctly measure the noise level existing at the point where the microphone is placed. The following steps must be taken successively:

- Batteries must be checked before use and during long measuring sessions.
- A wind shield must be used if the air velocity is noticeable. It should anyway be used all the time as a dust shield.
- The microphone should be oriented as described previously.
- All intruding objects such as the body of the sound level meter (SLM) or the operator itself will degrade the frequency response of the microphone at high frequencies and directivity effects will appear at much smaller frequencies. Therefore, the SLM should be, whenever possible, installed on a stable and sturdy tripod equipped with resilient blocks to isolate the sound level meter from vibration and consequent spurious readings. The operator should be at a reasonable distance (2-3 m) behind the sound level metert. Extension cables should be used if possible when measurements are to be made in a restricted area. When the instrument makes it possible, an extension rod should be used for the microphone. For walk-through surveys, the SLM should be held well away from the body.
- The SLM must be calibrated before any measuring session using a calibrator described in Section 6.8. If the temperature of the instrument is significantly different from the ambient temperature where it will be used, it should be first warmed up before calibration and use. The calibration must be checked at the end of the session. If the instrument is not calibrated anymore, the data might have to be discarded and the reasons for this calibration change should be investigated as this might indicate an important malfunctioning of the instrument.
- Nowadays, it is much more advantageous to use an integrating sound level meter to determine the $L_{Aeq,T}$ over a representative period of time T than to use a simple SLM on fast or slow giving an instantaneous value.

Noise Dosimeter

In recent decades, increased mechanisation has drastically changed the industrial work environment. This has led to many changes to an employee's work pattern. It used to be the case on the majority of production lines that an employee would stay in one place for their working shift. Therefore, monitoring their noise exposure with a sound level meter was very straightforward. However, with the increase in completely mechanised production lines, employees may now supervise several automated machines. This means that they now move around from area to area resulting in much more dramatic and varied exposure to noise.

A noise dosimeter is a small, light device that clips to a person's belt with a small microphone that fastens to the person's collar, close to an ear. The dosimeter stores the noise level information and carries out an averaging process. It is useful in industry where noise usually varies in duration and intensity, and where the person changes locations.

A noise dosimeter requires the following settings:

(a) Criterion Level: exposure limit for 8 hours per day five days per week. Criterion level is 85 dB(A) for many jurisdictions, 90 dB(A) for Quebec and 87 dB(A) for Canadian federal jurisdictions. Find out more about the exposure levels in the OSH Answers document Noise - Occupational Exposure Limits in Canada).

(b) Exchange rate: 3 dB or 5 dB as specified in the noise regulation.

(c) Threshold: noise level limit below which the dosimeter does not accumulate noise dose data.

Wearing the dosimeter over a complete work shift gives the average noise exposure or noise dose for that person. This is usually expressed as a noise exposure level, $L_{ex,T}$. This is a logarithm which takes into account the exposure and the actual time worked. In the past, it was often expressed as a percentage of the maximum permitted exposure. If a person has received a noise dose of 100% over a work shift, this means that the average noise exposure is at the maximum permitted. For example, with a criterion level of 90 dB(A) and an exchange rate of 3 dB(A), an eight-hour exposure to 90 dB(A) gives a 100% dose. A four-hour exposure to 93 dB(A) is also a 100% dose, whereas an eight-hour exposure to 93 dB(A) is a noise dose of 200%.

Usually the manufacturer electronically adjusts dosimeters to the criterion level and exchange rate in use. You may have to adjust them to suit the exposure guidelines/standards in force in your jurisdiction.

Dosimeters also give an equivalent sound or noise level. This is the average exposure level for noise over the time dosimeter was on. It has the same total sound energy as the actual, variable sound levels to which a person is exposed over the same time period. Scientific evidence suggests that hearing loss is affected by the total noise energy exposure. If a person is exposed over an eight-hour work shift to varying noise levels, it is possible to calculate an equivalent sound level which would equal the same total sound energy exposure. This would have the same effect on the person's hearing as the variable exposure actually received.

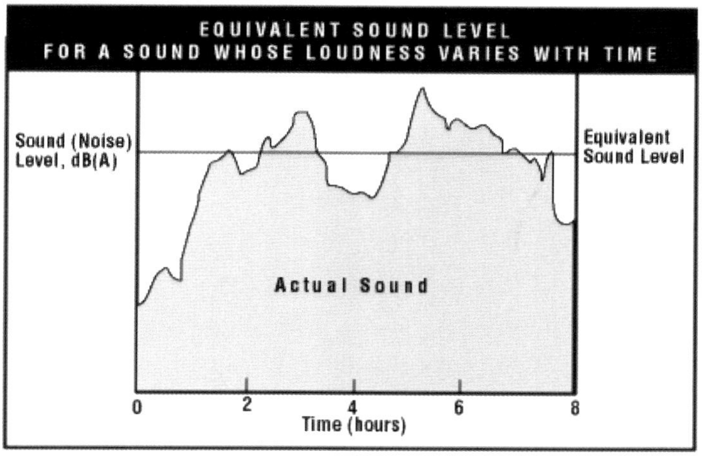

The shaded area under the line that shows how the sound level changes over time (the "curve") represents the total sound exposure over eight hours.

With innovations in digital technology, noise dosimeters are becoming smaller and smaller. The latest "badge" dosimeters have certain advantages over traditional dosimeters. Because the dosimeter is small and light enough to be worn on the shoulder, it means there are no cumbersome microphone cables. If there are no cables to get in the way, not only is it safer to wear, but also employees are less resistant to wearing it and much more likely to forget it is there. This means the quality of the noise data collected will be improved.

Because of the small size of badge-type products, it is also possible to mount them in more innovative ways, such as on a hard hat, close to the ear, without interfering with an employee's working process in any way. This allows the dosimeter to not be mounted on clothing at all, therefore completely removing it from the employee's mind.

Standards and Accuracy

Noise dosimeters are manufactured to IEC 61252, the international standard for dosimeters. IEC 61252 "Type 2" regulations require a field calibrator of a dosimeter before each use. Field calibrators produce a noise signal, normally a tone of 1 KHz at 114 dB. It is best practice to run the calibration test after any period of field measurement, as well, to check that there has been no significant drift of the dosimeter during the measurement.

The dosimeter and the acoustic calibrator must be returned to the manufacturer for a full calibration every two years for a true calibration. A lab conducts a battery of tests, including testing measurements across all frequencies and levels to ensure the dosimeter still meets the requirements of IEC 61652.

The Post Process

Dosimeters measure all essential parameters for workplace noise regulations such as daily exposures and peak levels. However, to serve a purpose this data must be easily accessible and be presented in a format that is comprehensible to someone not familiar with acoustic terminology. Modern software will give the dosimeter user the ability to store data in a format that accounts for who was being measured, when these measurements were taken, and at what workstation. Software today can output data into reports automatically, including the average and peak time history, in a simplified format with all required data for workplace noise regulations.

In conclusion, dosimeters are crucial in noise monitoring in today's modern working environment, with its highly mobile workers and varying noise exposure. Dosimeters provide valuable information by using logged time history data that show exactly when and where specific noise exposure took place. These details allow the implementation of proper controls to prevent hearing damage, which is the true end goal of any noise survey.

Equal-loudness Contour

The ear is not equally sensitive to all frequencies, particularly in the low and high frequency ranges. The response to frequencies over the entire audio range has been charted, originally by Fletcher and Munson in 1933, with later revisions by other authors, as a set of curves showing the sound pressure levels of pure tones that are perceived as being equally loud. The curves are plotted for each 10 dB rise in level with the reference tone being at 1 kHz. Also called *loudness level contours* and the *Fletcher-Munson curves.*

The curves are lowest in the range from 1 to 5 kHz, with a dip at 4 kHz, indicating that the ear is most sensitive to frequencies in this range. The intensity level of higher or lower tones must be raised substantially in order to create the same impression of loudness. The phon scale was devised to express this subjective impression of loudness, since the decibel scale alone refers to actual sound pressure or sound intensity levels.

Historically, the A, B, and C weighting networks on a sound level meter were derived as the inverse of the 40, 70 and 100 dB Fletcher-Munson curves and used to determine sound level.

The lowest curve repesents the threshol of hearing , the highest the threshol of pain.

Fletcher Munson Curve

The Fletcher Munson Curve is the first of several measurements that came to be called *equal-loudness contours.* These contours are visual diagrams displaying the effect that loudness and frequency has on human hearing.

With all of the focus on the frequency response of diaphragms and mechanisms that reproduce sound, such as speakers and acoustic environments, nobody considered the biological organs that perceive sound. The aforenamed scientists considered the problem on a higher order and measured the influence the human ear has on perceiving volume, pitch, and the relative loudness level of each frequency range compared to one another. He then launched one of the earliest studies in psychoacoustics ever.

Below is a large sized image of the Fletcher Munson diagram including all of the reported data.

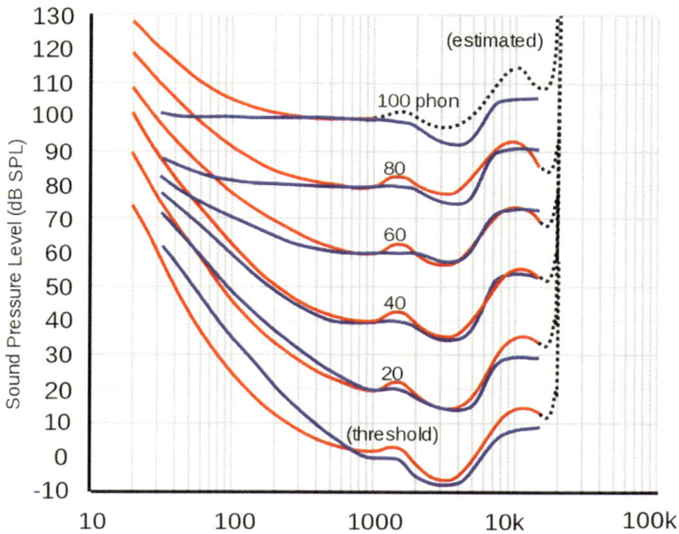

Equal-loudness contours (red) (from ISO 226:2003 revision)
Fletcher–Munson curves shown (blue) for comparison

The blue lines are the data reported in the original research. The red lines follow the measurements by Robinson and Dadson, which we'll discuss next, that ultimately become the current equal loudness contour international standard. Both are plotted logarithmically on the horizontal access across the frequency spectrum of human hearing. On the vertical access are sound pressure levels from -10 dB up to 130 dB, allowing us to see six sets of measurements at once at 20 dB increments.

The dip between 3 kHz and 4 kHz correlates to the increased sensitivity of the human ear in that range, as mentioned above. A slight increase of 2 dB to 5 dB occurs between 1 kHz and 2 kHz, while an even greater sensitivity appears linearly up between 4 kHz and 11 kHz. This is an inverse relationship, which means these regions require less loudness for humans to perceive them as being the same volume as louder frequencies.

Note that while the two sets of curves are relatively similar above 500 Hz, they differ quite drastically in the bass and sub-bass regions. It's accepted that the Robinson

Dadson Curve is more accurate, although the original curve continued to relate more closely to all other standards all the way until the ISO 226 standard was adjusted in 2003. The discrepancies in the bass and sub-bass frequency ranges have been attempted to be explained away, yet no explanation has been deemed satisfactory, by saying:

- The measuring devices weren't properly calibrated for those regions
- The judging criteria has changed over the years, varying for different frequencies
- The subjects were suffering from over-exposure to low-frequency sounds before testing
- The race of the participants had an effect (inclusion of Japanese data)

Any proper experiment that has been accepted as an international standard will have controlled for listener fatigue, so we can rule that out. It's important to note that sub-bass frequencies are felt more than heard, so that's partially why this discrepancy has been glossed over.

Robinson Dadson Curve

Various standards had been accepted in the time between the original report and that of Robinson and Dadson. The latter's published data varied more significantly from the time's current standard and average of other results than did any other. Fortunately, the original 40-phon measurement, which was the basis for the A-weighting standard, agreed quite well with the Robinson Dadson 40-phon measurement (as seen above in the figure), which brought confidence for the rest of the measurements.

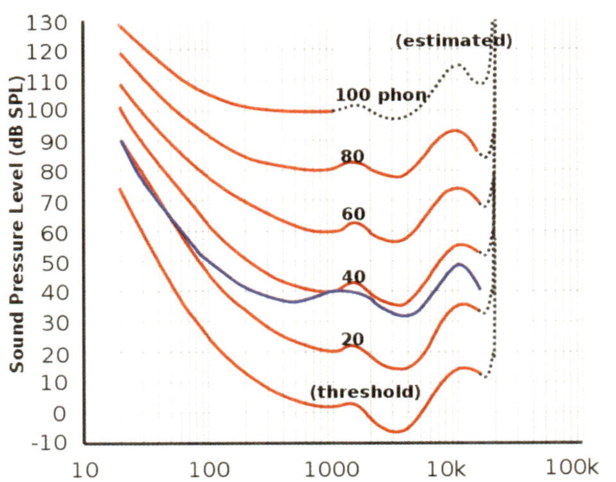

Equal-loudness contours (red) (from ISO 226:2003 revisi
Original ISO standard shown (blue) for 40-phons

Above are the current standards, the ISO 226 standard based on Robinson and Dadson's reported data, but adjusted using recent assessments by researchers across the globe in 2003. The blue line is the original ISO standard for 40-phons, which is not to be confused with the original 40-phon curve. The adjustments, to everyone's relief, brought the data back into reconciliation with the data from the initial paper, especially in the bass regions.

This is currently deemed the most accurate measurement and is used internationally by all professionals, despite the questionably fluctuating results in the bass and sub-bass frequency ranges.

Equal Loudness Contours: Methodology

We've focused on the results, but how does an equal loudness curve get measured? We can't rely on self-reporting by listeners because subjective data can't be objectively compared. So how is a human hearing curve built?

The basic methodology is the playing of two pure tones using sine waves at set frequencies and at incremented sound pressure levels (volumes) while having a listener report when they perceive the two as being at equal volumes.

The participants must be an average youth with no significant hearing loss. Any reported hearing impairment disqualifies a person from the experiment.

It has been determined that the human auditory system can perceive frequencies from around 20 Hz up to around 22 kHz. The maximum of 22 kHz in young people is lowered to around 20 kHz in adults. As we begun to understand resonances of cavities, researchers figured there would be peaks and nulls in the frequency response due to the shape and length of the ear canal and even in the functionality of the middle ear. They were right.

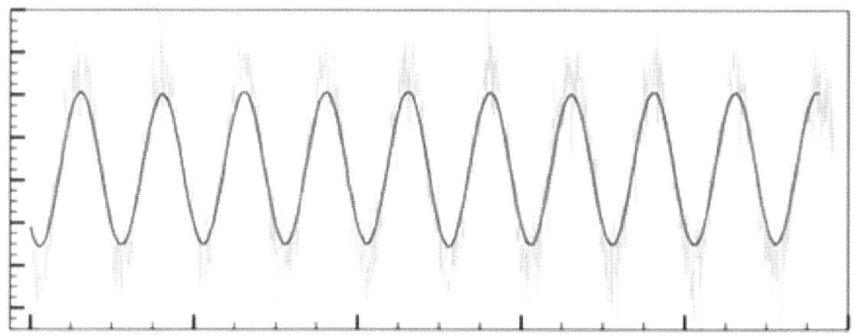

A pure tone sine wave shown over one with a more natural timber

The first measurements reported in the *Loudness* paper used a reference tone of 1000 Hz, which was fluctuated in volume until the participant said it was the same volume as the experimental tone. They repeated this for the entire frequency range of human hearing across many participants and averaged the results. The test was performed at the absolute threshold of hearing (very quiet) and incremented at 10 dB until reaching the threshold of pain (very loud).

Researchers Churcher and King attempted a second set of measurements in 1937 but were so far off the currently accepted mark that their results were ultimately disregarded. It was in 1956 that Robinson and Dadson's results were published using the same methodology but a more granular and meticulous approach.

Side vs. Frontal Presentation using Headphones vs. Loudspeakers

The Robinson-Dadson team used headphones with their participants while the Fletcher-Munson team used loudspeakers in front of the participants. There are two key differences here:

- Side versus frontal presentation of sound
- The distance of the human ear from the sound source

Headphones offer a purely side presentation of sound from a very close distance from the sound source, while loudspeakers are at a much greater distance from a more realistic angle when considering reflections in a room and in nature. The differences in the bass measurements were attempted to be explained away by the use of headphones but the ISO report says the team used 'compensated headphones.' To this day, we aren't sure what that even means, so again it's another inconclusive excuse.

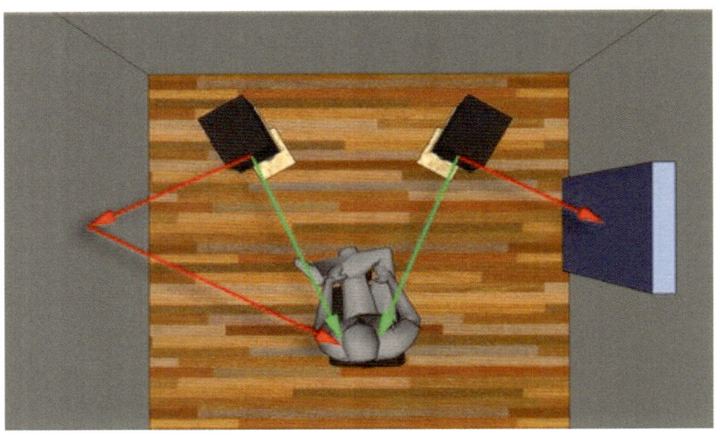

The problem of acoustics, removed by headphones or acoustic treatment

Headphones can also offer a very flat frequency response without needing acoustic treatment in the environment like loudspeakers will. This means they dodge all of the issues of constructive and deconstructive interference due to the box-shaped room. They also avoid issues related to the shape of the ear and head and how these influence certain frequencies based on the angle at which the sound comes towards the head.

At the end of the day, no matter which method a research team uses, the other way of listening still exists and is in widespread use by listeners every day. Perhaps the best approach would be to maintain two sets of standards, one for studio headphones and one for studio monitors, while providing an averaged summation of the two to professionals.

The Implications for Professional Mixing & Mastering Engineers

In the most simple manner of reducing all of this down to a bite-sized explanation:

If a mix is left unchanged with its tonal balance left alone, it will sound different at lower volumes and at higher volumes. At the lowest volumes, the bass and upper frequency ranges will be much quieter than the mid-range. At high volumes, bass will be more present, high frequencies can become too forward, and the mid-range will more or less remain the same with slight variance.

So how do we deal with this problem as a mastering or mixing engineer? How do we achieve a pleasing balance of frequencies for the listener no matter what volume they choose to enjoy our music or movies at?

Newcomers to the field of mixing will become extremely frustrated as they check their mixes at varying volumes, boosting and cutting and doing and un-doing the same changes over and over again, not understanding the impact of the findings in the original loudness curves.

It makes sense to say "Well, we should just mix at loud volumes, since that's when our listener's are paying the most attention anyways. If they want background noise they turn the music down anyways." It does make sense, accept you'll end up with ear fatigue and not be able to make rational decisions during a lengthy mix session.

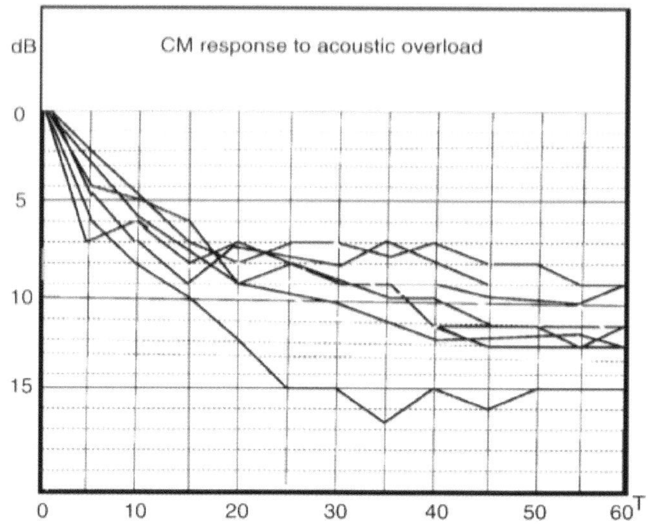

We begin to experience ear fatigue with extended acoustic overload

What we need to do is mix at an average, comfortable volume for the bulk of the progress, preferably in the range of 80 to 85 dB SPL. You need a calibrated mixing level that you always return to and come to know better than any other volume. After this, we should use our studio monitors and studio subwoofer to make adjustments at a higher volume. This is when we'll make slight adjustments to faders, within the range of 2 dB to 5 dB and nothing more drastic. This is when we should listen critically and make some adjustments on our equalizers. Don't keep the volume high for long. Reduce the gain and check again at an average volume and make sure it still sounds great there.

Finally, we should drop the volume to a lower amount and reference our mix on our mixing headphones. We should expect the bass and upper frequencies to be slightly more quiet than they were, relatively, but they should still sound great. If you choose to make adjustments here, make them even slighter than you did at high volumes, because what you do here will be multiplied by two or three as you boost the volume back up.

Don't try to compensate for what consumers do. They already have their own solutions. For instance, we buy subwoofers so we can still hear the bass on our favorite songs and movies at normal volumes. Our stereos have bass boost buttons to help compensate at low volumes. If you try to compensate first, then there will be double compensation and too much bass! Your goal is always to produce the best result in the flattest frequency response environment possible. This minimizes all potential problems as much as possible once the audio is distributed to the masses.

You may need to repeat the mixing procedure above two or three times with tinier and tinier changes until you reach a middle ground where the mix sounds fantastic at an average-to-high volume and still sounds very good a very high volume and a low volume. Don't drive yourself nuts though. No mixer or mastering engineer can overcome the nature of how humans perceive hearing at different volumes. Your goal is to minimize the difference as much as possible by achieving a pleasing mix at all volumes. This mix might sound slightly different at varying volumes, but it is pleasing nonetheless.

Noise Map

A Noise Map is a map of an area which is coloured according to the noise levels in the area. Sometimes, the noise levels may be shown by contour lines which show the boundaries between different noise levels in an area.

The noise levels over an area will be varying all the time. For example, noise levels may rise as a vehicle approaches, and reduce again after it has passed. This would cause a short-term variations in noise level. In the slightly longer term, noise levels may be higher in peak periods when the roads are busy, and lower in off-peak periods. Then again, there is a greater volume of activity from more people and traffic in the day-time than in the evening or at night. In the longer term, wind, weather and season all affect noise levels.

This means that it is not possible to say with confidence what the noise level will be at any particular point at any instant in time, but where the noise sources are well-defined, such as road or rail traffic, or aircraft, then it is possible to say with some confidence what the long-term average noise level will be.

It may be thought that the best way of doing this is by measurement, but experience shows that this is not the case. For a start, a long-term average must be measured over a long period of time. Secondly, to obtain complete coverage of an area, measurements would have to be made on private property, where access might be difficult, and thirdly, measurements cannot distinguish the different sources of noise, so they would not be able to give information on how much noise was being made by each of the sources in an area.

For these and other reasons, noise mapping is usually done by calculation based on a computerised noise model of an area, although measurements may be appropriate in some cases.

A further benefit of having a noise model is that it can be used to assess the effects of transportation and other plans. Thus the effect of a proposed new road can be assessed and suitable noise mitigation can be designed to minimise its impact. This is particularly important in noise action planning, where a cost-benefit analysis of various options can be tested before a decision is made.

Strategic Noise Maps

A strategic noise map is designed to assess noise exposure in a given area, resulting from particular noise sources such as roads, railways and airports. Such maps are normally prepared using computer modelling techniques. Such techniques calculate the noise level at specific points resulting from the sound emanating from the source being studied. The modelling software uses source data such as traffic flow, type of road and rail, types of vehicles and speeds.

In accordance with the requirements of the Noise Directive the EPA has made available the strategic noise mapping of major agglomeration airports, major roads and major rail networks, in the form of noise contours for the L_{den} (day, evening, night) and L_{night} (night) periods. A noise map is a graphical representation of the predicted situation with regards to noise in a particular area with different colours representing different noise levels in decibels.

All noise maps are presented in terms of two noise indicators: L_{den} and L_{night}.

- L_{den} is the day-evening-night noise indicator and it represents the noise indicator for overall annoyance. It is 'weighted' to account for extra annoyance in the evening and night periods. The END defines an L_{den} threshold of 55 dB for reporting on the numbers of people exposed.
- L_{night} is the night time noise indicator and is used in the assessment of sleep disturbance. An L_{night} threshold of 50 dB is defined for reporting on the numbers of people exposed.

Noise Measurement

Sound (Noise) Level

Sound and unwanted sound, called noise, is the result of fluctuations or oscillations in atmospheric pressure. These excite the ear mechanism and evoke the sensation of hearing.

The human ear responds to changes in sound pressure over a very wide range - the loudest sound pressure to which the human ear responds is ten million times greater than the softest. This large ratio is reduced to a more manageable size by the use of logarithms. The logarithms scale provides a more convenient way of comparing the sound pressure of one sound with another. To avoid a scale which is too compressed, a factor of 10 is introduced, giving rise to the decibel unit.

The level of sound pressure p is said to be Lp decibels greater than a reference sound pressure Pref according to the following definition:

Sound Pressure Level (Lp or SPL) $= 10 \log_{10}(P^2 / Pref^2)$ dB

$= 20 \log_{10}P - 20\log_{10}Pref$ dB

where p is the sound pressure fluctuation (above or below atmospheric pressure) and Pref is 20 micropascals (2×10^{-5}Pa), which is approximately the threshold of hearing.

The decibel scale is shown in.

The Decibel Scale

The Decibel Scale - some typical sound levels

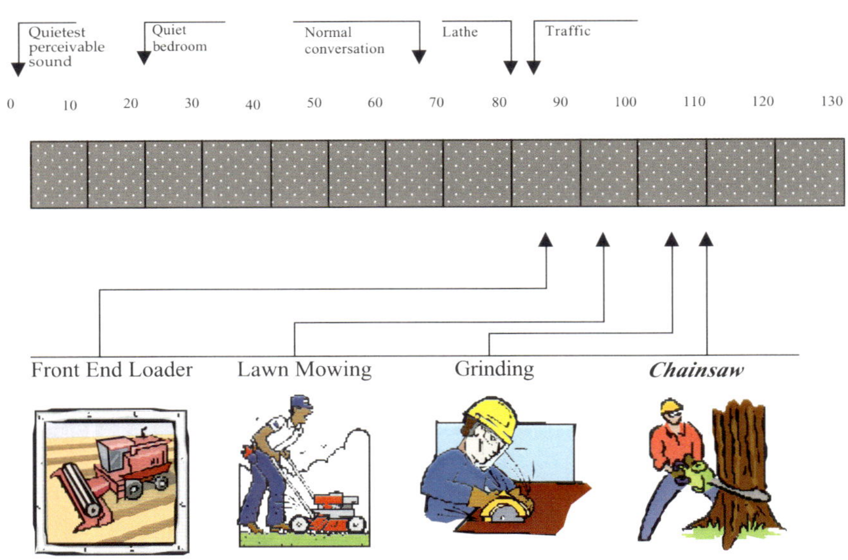

A-weighted Decibels, dBA

The threshold of human hearing varies with frequency, being most sensitive to sound mid frequencies (500 Hz to 4000 Hz), and less sensitive at lower and higher frequencies. The pressure amplitude of a sound therefore does not directly relate to its perceived loudness and both frequency and amplitude need to be taken into account. For low level sounds, a filter having a frequency response corresponding to that of human hearing (in level range about 40 dBA), is incorporated in sound level meters. Sound level measurements made using this filter (A-weighting) are described as A-weighted decibels, dBA.

The level of a sound expressed in dBA is a reasonable measure of the loudness of that sound. Different sounds having the same dBA level generally sound about equally as loud, although the character of the noise also plays a part in its perceived loudness.

A change of 1dBA or less in the level of a sound is difficult for most people to detect, whilst a 3 dBA to 5dBA change corresponds to small but noticeable change in loudness. A 10 dBA change is generally accepted to correspond to an approximate doubling or halving in loudness. Table following, gives examples of dBA levels are shown in table.

Table: Example Noise Levels

Sound Pressure Level (dBA)	Typical Source	Subjective Evaluation
140 130 120 110	Long range gun, gunner s ear Threshold of pain Jet take-off at 100m Night club dance floor	Extremely noisy to intolerable
100 90	Loud car hom at 3 metres Heavy truck at 10m	Very noisy
80 70	Curbside of busy street Car interior	Loud
60 50	Normal conversation at 1m Office noise	Moderate to quiet
40 30	Living room in quiet area Inside bedroom at night	Quiet to very quiet
20	Unoccupied recording studio	Almost silent

Statistical Analysis of Sound (Noise)

Ambient sound varies in level over time and so is commonly described statistically in terms of exceedence levels. These levels summarise the percentage of time a noise level was exceeded during the measurement period at the measurement point.

For example, if a noise level of 80 dBA was exceeded 10% of the time during a sampling period, this result would be described as an LA10 of 80 dBA. Statistical sound level meters usually generate a range of percentile results between 0 and 100.

An A-weighted noise level exceeded for N% of a given measurement period is denoted as an LAN of that level. LA1 is the noise level exceeded for 1% of the time, LA10 the noise exceeded for 10% of the time, and so on. LA90 is a commonly used measure of the average minimum or background A-weighted noise level.

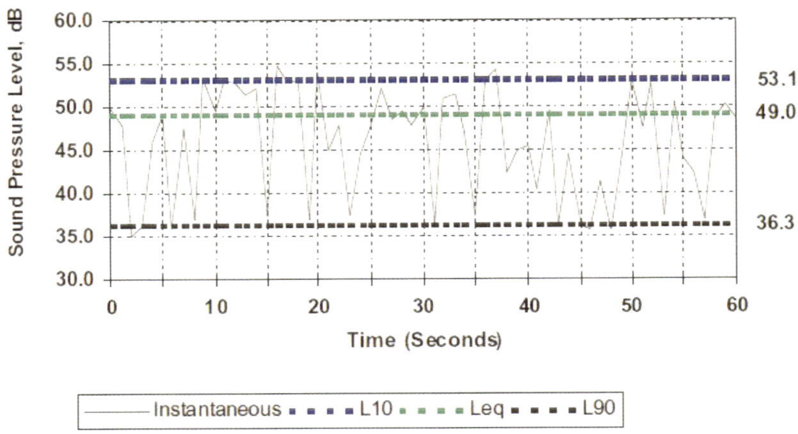

Sound Variation with Time and its Descriptors

Another index of sound level that is also in common usage is the A-weighted equivalent continuous noise level, denoted as LAeq . LAeq is essentially the constant sound pressure level, which is equivalent to (contains the same amount of acoustical energy as) the varying sounds level over the measurement period.

depicts a sixty second measurement sample of a varying sound and some of the descriptors discussed.

References

- Viemeister NF, Plack CJ (1993). Human Psychophysics. Springer Handbook of Auditory Research. Springer, New York, NY. pp. 116–154. doi:10.1007/978-1-4612-2728-1_4. ISBN 978-1-4612-7644-9
- Soundlevelmeters: explainthatstuff.com, Retrieved 25 June 2018
- Kates JM, Arehart KH (April 2005). "Coherence and the speech intelligibility index". The Journal of the Acoustical Society of America. 117 (4 Pt 1): 2224–37. PMID 15898663
- Audiometer, meniere-s-disease-cure: menieresdisease-treatment.com, Retrieved 19 June 2018
- Moore BC (2014-05-04). Auditory Processing of Temporal Fine Structure: Effects of Age and Hearing Loss. New Jersey: World Scientific Publishing Company. ISBN 9789814579650
- Visual-reinforcement-audiometry, specialty-centers-and-programs treatments-and-services, ear-nose-and-throat, specialties-services: childrens.com, Retrieved 25 May 2018

- Shamma S, Lorenzi C (May 2013). "On the balance of envelope and temporal fine structure in the encoding of speech in the early auditory system". The Journal of the Acoustical Society of America. 133 (5): 2818–33. doi:10.1121/1.4795783. PMC 3663870. PMID 23654388
- Profession, focus-on-audiometry-a-bit-of-history-2148: audiology-worldnews.com, Retrieved 30 May 2018
- International Electrotechnical Commission, IEC. "IEC 61672-1:2013 Electroacoustics - Sound level meters - Part 1: Specifications". iec.ch. Retrieved 2018-03-16
- Audiology: healthline.com, Retrieved 3 July 2018
- Goldsworthy RL, Greenberg JE (December 2004). "Analysis of speech-based Speech Transmission Index methods with implications for nonlinear operations". The Journal of the Acoustical Society of America. 116 (6): 3679–89. PMID 15658718
- Profession, focus-on-audiometry-a-bit-of-history-2148: audiology-worldnews.com, Retrieved 30 May 2018
- Depireux DA, Elhilali M, eds. (2014-01-15). Handbook of Modern Techniques in Auditory Cortex (first ed.). Nova Science Pub Inc. ISBN 9781628088946

4

Hearing Loss and Disorders

Hearing loss or hearing impairment is the partial or complete inability to hear. It can be temporary or permanent and can occur in one or both ears. Hearing loss can be of different kinds, such as sensorineural hearing loss, nonsyndromic deafness, unilateral hearing loss, etc. This chapter discusses in detail the different kinds of hearing disorders, such as Ménière's disease, tinnitus, hyperacusis and musical ear syndrome.

Hearing Loss

Hearing loss is when your ability to hear is reduced. A hearing loss makes it more difficult for you to hear speech and other sounds.

The most common causes of hearing loss are noise and ageing. In most cases a hearing loss cannot be cured. Hearing loss is typically treated with hearing aids.

Hearing loss can be temporary or permanent. It often comes on gradually as you get older, but it can sometimes happen suddenly.

While there are different types of hearing loss, presbycusis (loss of hearing that occurs gradually as one ages) is the most common for those 55 and older. Exposure to loud noises also contributes to many with hearing damage. Genetics, birth defects, infections of the head or ear, excessive earwax (temporary hearing loss issue), and reactions to drugs are all triggers for hearing loss. While you cannot reverse most types of hearing loss, there are options to improve your hearing.

Signs and Symptoms of Hearing Loss

It's not always easy to tell if you're losing your hearing.

Common signs include:

- difficulty hearing other people clearly, and misunderstanding what they say, especially in noisy places
- asking people to repeat themselves
- listening to music or watching television loudly

- having to concentrate hard to hear what other people are saying, which can be tiring or stressful

The signs can be slightly different if you only have hearing loss in 1 ear or if a young child has hearing loss.

Hearing Loss Statistics

- About 20 percent of Americans, 48 million, report some degree of hearing loss.
- At age 65, one out of three people has a hearing loss.
- 60 percent of the people with hearing loss are either in the work force or in educational settings.
- While people in the workplace with the mildest hearing losses show little or no drop in income compared to their normal hearing peers, as the hearing loss increases, so does the reduction in compensation.
- About 2-3 of every 1,000 children in the United States are born with a detectable hearing loss in one or both ears.
- Almost 15 percent of school children (ages 6-19) have some degree of hearing loss.

Use of the terms "hearing impaired", "deaf-mute", or "deaf and dumb" to describe deaf and hard of hearing people is discouraged by advocacy organizations as they are offensive to many deaf and hard of hearing people.

- Hearing loss exists when there is diminished sensitivity to the sounds normally heard. The terms hearing impaired or hard of hearing are usually reserved for people who have relative insensitivity to sound in the speech frequencies. The severity of a hearing loss is categorized according to the increase in volume above the usual level necessary before the listener can detect it.
- Deafness is defined as a degree of loss such that a person is unable to understand speech even in the presence of amplification. In profound deafness, even the loudest sounds produced by an audiometer (an instrument used to measure hearing by producing pure tone sounds through a range of frequencies) may not be detected. In total deafness, no sounds at all, regardless of amplification or method of production, are heard.
- Speech perception – Another aspect of hearing involves the perceived clarity of a word rather than the amplitude of sound made by the word. In humans, that aspect is usually measured by tests of speech perception. These tests measure one's ability to understand speech, not to merely detect sound. There are very rare types of hearing loss which affect speech perception alone.

Hearing Standards

Human hearing extends in frequency from 20–20,000 Hz, and in amplitude from 0 dB to 130 dB or more. 0 dB does not represent absence of sound, but rather the softest sound an average unimpaired human ear can hear; some people can hear down to −5 or even −10 dB. 130 dB represents the threshold of pain. But the ear doesn't hear all frequencies equally well; hearing sensitivity peaks around 3000 Hz. There are many qualities of human hearing besides frequency range and amplitude that can't easily be measured quantitatively. But for many practical purposes, normative hearing is defined by a frequency versus amplitude graph, or audiogram, charting sensitivity thresholds of hearing at defined frequencies. Because of the cumulative impact of age and exposure to noise and other acoustic insults, 'typical' hearing may not be normative.

Causes

Hearing loss has multiple causes, including ageing, genetics, perinatal problems and acquired causes like noise and disease. For some kinds of hearing loss the cause may be classified as of unknown cause.

Age

There is a progressive loss of ability to hear high frequencies with aging known as presbycusis. For men, this can start as early as 25 and women at 30. Although genetically variable it is a normal concomitant of ageing and is distinct from hearing losses caused by noise exposure, toxins or disease agents. Common conditions that can increase the risk of hearing loss in elderly people are high blood pressure, diabetes or the use of certain medications harmful to the ear. While everyone loses hearing with age, the amount and type of hearing loss is variable.

Noise

Noise exposure is the cause of approximately half of all cases of hearing loss, causing some degree of problems in 5% of the population globally. The National Institute for Occupational Safety and Health (NIOSH) recognizes that the majority of hearing loss is not due to age, but due to noise exposure. By correcting for age in assessing hearing, one tends to overestimate the hearing loss due to noise for some and underestimate it for others.

Hearing loss due to noise may be temporary, called a 'temporary threshold shift', a reduced sensitivity to sound over a wide frequency range resulting from exposure to a brief but very loud noise like a gunshot, firecracker, jet engine, jackhammer, etc. or to exposure to loud sound over a few hours such as during a pop concert or nightclub session. Recovery of hearing is usually within 24 hours, but may take up to a week. Both constant exposure to loud sounds (85 dB(A) or above) and one-time exposure to extremely loud sounds (120 dB(A) or above) may cause permanent hearing loss.

Noise-induced hearing loss (NIHL) typically manifests as elevated hearing thresholds (i.e. less sensitivity or muting) between 3000 and 6000 Hz, centered at 4000 Hz. As noise damage progresses, damage spreads to affect lower and higher frequencies. On an audiogram, the resulting configuration has a distinctive notch, called a 'noise' notch. As aging and other effects contribute to higher frequency loss (6–8 kHz on an audiogram), this notch may be obscured and entirely disappear.

Various governmental, industry and standards organizations set noise standards.

The U.S. Environmental Protection Agency has identified the level of 70 dB(A) (40% louder to twice as loud as normal conversation; typical level of TV, radio, stereo; city street noise) for 24hour exposure as the level necessary to protect the public from hearing loss and other disruptive effects from noise, such as sleep disturbance, stress-related problems, learning detriment, etc. Noise levels are typically in the 65 to 75 dB (A) range for those living near airports of freeways and may result in hearing damage if sufficient time is spent outdoors.

Louder sounds cause damage in a shorter period of time. Estimation of a "safe" duration of exposure is possible using an *exchange rate* of 3 dB. As 3 dB represents a doubling of intensity of sound, duration of exposure must be cut in half to maintain the same energy dose. For workplace noise regulation, the "safe" daily exposure amount at 85 dB A, known as an exposure action value, is 8 hours, while the "safe" exposure at 91 dB(A) is only 2 hours. Different standards use exposure action values between 80dBA and 90dBA. Note that for some people, sound may be damaging at even lower levels than 85 dB A. Exposures to other ototoxins (such as pesticides, some medications including chemotherapy agents, solvents, etc.) can lead to greater susceptibility to noise damage, as well as causing its own damage. This is called a *synergistic* interaction. Since noise damage is cumulative over long periods of time, persons who are exposed to non-workplace noise, like recreational activities or environmental noise, may have compounding damage from all sources.

Some national and international organizations and agencies use an exchange rate of 4 dB or 5 dB. While these exchange rates may indicate a wider zone of comfort or safety, they can significantly underestimate the damage caused by loud noise. For example, at 100 dB (nightclub music level), a 3 dB exchange rate would limit exposure to 15 minutes; the 5 dB exchange rate allows an hour.

Many people are unaware of the presence of environmental sound at damaging levels, or of the level at which sound becomes harmful. Common sources of damaging noise levels include car stereos, children's toys, motor vehicles, crowds, lawn and maintenance equipment, power tools, gun use, musical instruments, and even hair dryers. Noise damage is cumulative; all sources of damage must be considered to assess risk. If one is exposed to loud sound (including music) at high levels or for extended durations (85 dB A or greater), then hearing loss will occur. Sound intensity (sound energy, or propensity to cause damage to the ears) increases dramatically with proximity according to an inverse square law: halving the distance to the sound quadruples the sound intensity.

In the USA, 12.5% of children aged 6–19 years have permanent hearing damage from excessive noise exposure. The World Health Organization estimates that half of those between 12 and 35 are at risk from using personal audio devices that are too loud.

Hearing loss due to noise has been described as primarily a condition of modern society. In preindustrial times, humans had far less exposure to loud sounds. Studies of primitive peoples indicate that much of what has been attributed to age-related hearing loss may be long term cumulative damage from all sources, especially noise. People living in preindustrial societies have considerably less hearing loss than similar populations living in modern society. Among primitive people who have migrated into modern society, hearing loss is proportional to the number of years spent in modern society. Military service in World War II, the Korean War, and the Vietnam War, has likely also caused hearing loss in large numbers of men from those generations, though proving that hearing loss was a direct result of military service is problematic without entry and exit audiograms.

Hearing loss in adolescents may be caused by loud noise from toys, music by headphones, and concerts or events. In 2017, the Centers for Disease Control and Prevention brought their researchers together with experts from the World Health Organization and academia to examine the risk of hearing loss from excessive noise exposure in and outside the workplace in different age groups, as well as actions being taken to reduce the burden of the condition. A summary report was published in 2018.

Genetic

Hearing loss can be inherited. Around 75–80% of all these cases are inherited by recessive genes, 20–25% are inherited by dominant genes, 1–2% are inherited by X-linked patterns, and fewer than 1% are inherited by mitochondrial inheritance.

When looking at the genetics of deafness, there are 2 different forms, syndromic and nonsyndromic. Syndromic deafness occurs when there are other signs or medical problems aside from deafness in an individual. This accounts for around 30% of deaf individuals who are deaf from a genetic standpoint. Nonsyndromic deafness occurs when there are no other signs or medical problems associated with an individual other than deafness. From a genetic standpoint, this accounts for the other 70% of cases, and represents the majority of hereditary hearing loss. Syndromic cases occur with diseases such as Usher syndrome, Stickler syndrome, Waardenburg syndrome, Alport's syndrome, and neurofibromatosis type 2. These are diseases that have deafness as one of the symptoms or as a common feature associated with it. Many of the genetic mutations giving rise to syndromic deafness have been identified. In nonsyndromic cases, where deafness is the only finding, it is more difficult to identify the genetic mutation although some have been discovered.

- Gene mapping has identified the genetic locations for several nonsyndromic dominant (DFNA#) and recessive (DFNB#) forms of deafness. The first gene mapped for non-syndromic deafness, DFNA1, involves a splice site mutation in the formin related homolog diaphanous 1 (DIAPH1). A single base change in a large Costa Rican family was identified as causative in a rare form of low frequency onset progressive hearing loss with autosomal dominant inheritance exhibiting variable age of onset and complete penetrance by age 30. The most common type of congenital hearing loss in developed countries is DFNB1, also known as connexin 26 deafness or GJB2-related deafness.
- The most common dominant syndromic forms of hearing loss include Stickler syndrome and Waardenburg syndrome.
- The most common recessive syndromic forms of hearing loss are Pendred syndrome and Usher syndrome.
- The congenital defect microtia, deformed or unformed outer ear, can be associated with partial or complete conductive deafness, depending upon the severity of the deformity and whether the middle ear is also affected. It can also be associated with abnormalities of the inner ear giving rise to an additional sensorineural component to the hearing loss (mixed deafness).
- Dozens of additional genes for nonsyndromic deafness have been identified.

Perinatal problems

- Fetal alcohol spectrum disorders are reported to cause hearing loss in up to 64% of infants born to alcoholic mothers, from the ototoxic effect on the developing fetus plus malnutrition during pregnancy from the excess alcohol intake.
- Premature birth can be associated with sensorineural hearing loss because of an increased risk of hypoxia, hyperbilirubinaemia, ototoxic medication and infection as well as noise exposure in the neonatal units. The risk of hearing loss is greatest for those weighing less than 1500 g at birth.

Disorders

- Strokes – Depending on what blood vessels are affected by the stroke, one of the symptoms can be deafness.
- Multiple sclerosis can have an effect on hearing as well. Multiple sclerosis, or MS, is an autoimmune disease where the immune system attacks the myelin sheath, a covering that protects the nerves. If the auditory nerve becomes damaged, the affected person will become completely deaf in one or both ears. There is no cure for MS.
- Perilymph fistula – a microtear in either the round or oval window (membranes

separating the middle and inner ear) of the cochlea causing perilymph to leak into the middle ear. This usually occurs as a consequence of trauma, including barotrauma, and can give rise to vertigo as well as hearing loss.

- Viral – viral infections of the ear can cause sensorineural hearing loss usually as the consequence of a labyrinthitis. The patient may be generally unwell at the time.
    - Measles may cause auditory nerve damage but usually gives rise to a chronic middle ear problem giving rise to a mixed hearing loss.
    - Mumps (Epidemic parotitis) may result in profound sensorineural hearing loss (90 dB or more), unilateral (one ear) or bilateral (both ears).
    - Congenital rubella (also called German measles) syndrome, can cause deafness in newborns.
    - Several varieties of herpes viruses that cause other diseases can also infect the ear, and can result in hearing loss: congenital infection with cytomegalovirus is responsible for deafness in newborn children and also progressive sensorineural hearing loss in childhood; herpes simplex type 1, oral herpes associated with cold sores; Epstein Barr virus that causes.
    - Mononucleosis; varicella zoster oticus that causes facial paralysis (Ramsay Hunt syndrome).
    - People with HIV/AIDS may develop hearing problems due to medications they take for the disease, the HIV virus, or due to an increased rate of other infections.
    - West Nile virus, which can cause a variety of neurological disorders, can also cause hearing loss by attacking the auditory nerve.
- Meningitis may damage the auditory nerve or the cochlea.
- Syphilis is commonly transmitted from pregnant women to their fetuses, and about a third of infected children will eventually become deaf.
- Inherited:
    - People with Down syndrome are more likely to have hearing loss. This is usually due to middle ear effusions in childhood but towards the end of the second decade they may develop a high frequency sensorineural hearing loss which can get progressively worse with time.
    - Charcot–Marie–Tooth disease variant 1E (CMT1E) is noted for demyelinating in addition to deafness.
    - Autoimmune disease is recognized as a cause for cochlear damage. Although rare, it is possible for autoimmune processes to target the cochlea specifical-

ly as a first presentation. Granulomatosis with polyangiitis is one of the autoimmune conditions that may precipitate hearing loss. Cogan's syndrome commonly presents with hearing loss.

- Otosclerosis is a condition that can cause fixation of the stapes (or stirrup) in the middle ear preventing its movement and causing a conductive hearing loss.
- Vestibular schwannoma, erroneously known as Acoustic neuromas, and other types of brain tumors can cause hearing loss by infringement of the tumor on the vestibulocochlear nerve.
- Congenital problems:
    - Superior semicircular canal dehiscence, a gap in the bone cover above the inner ear, can lead to low-frequency conductive hearing loss, autophony and vertigo.
- Recurring ear infections or concommitant secondary infections (such as bacterial infection subsequent to viral infection) can result in hearing loss.

Medications

Some medications may reversibly affect hearing. These medications are considered ototoxic. This includes loop diuretics such as furosemide and bumetanide, non-steroidal anti-inflammatory drugs (NSAIDs) both over-the-counter (aspirin, ibuprofen, naproxen) as well as prescription (celecoxib, diclofenac, etc.), paracetamol, quinine, and macrolide antibiotics. The link between NSAIDs and hearing loss tends to be greater in women, especially those who take ibuprofen six or more times a week. Others may cause permanent hearing loss. The most important group is the aminoglycosides (main member gentamicin) and platinum based chemotherapeutics such as cisplatin and carboplatin.

On October 18, 2007, the U.S. Food and Drug Administration (FDA) announced that a warning about possible sudden hearing loss would be added to drug labels of PDE5 inhibitors, which are used for erectile dysfunction.

Audiologic monitoring for ototoxicity allows for:

(1) Early detection of changes to hearing status presumably attributed to a drug/treatment regime so that changes in the drug regimen may be considered,

(2) Audiologic intervention when handicapping hearing impairment has occurred.

Co-administration of anti-oxidants and ototoxic medications may limit the extent of the ototoxic damage.

Chemicals

In addition to medications, hearing loss can also result from specific chemicals in the environment: metals, such as lead; solvents, such as toluene (found in crude oil, gasoline and automobile exhaust, for example); and asphyxiants. Combined with noise, these ototoxic chemicals have an additive effect on a person's hearing loss.

Hearing loss due to chemicals starts in the high frequency range and is irreversible. It damages the cochlea with lesions and degrades central portions of the auditory system. For some ototoxic chemical exposures, particularly styrene, the risk of hearing loss can be higher than being exposed to noise alone. The effects is greatest when the combined exposure include impulse noise.

- Solvents
  - toluene, styrene, xylene, *n*-hexane, ethyl benzene, white spirits/Stoddard, carbon disulfide, jet fuel, perchloroethylene, trichloroethylene, *p*-xylene
- Asphyxiants
  - carbon monoxide, hydrogen cyanide
- Heavy metals
  - lead, mercury, cadmium, arsenic, tin-hydrocarbon compounds (trimethyltin)
- Pesticides and herbicides – The evidence is weak regarding association between herbicides and hearing loss; hearing loss in such circumstances may be due to concommitant exposure to insecticides.
  - paraquat, organophosphates

A 2018 informational bulletin by the US Occupational Safety and Health Administration (OSHA) and the National Institute for Occupational Safety and Health (NIOSH) introduces the issue, provides examples of ototoxic chemicals, lists the industries and occupations at risk and provides prevention information.

Physical Trauma

There can be damage either to the ear itself or to the brain centers that process the aural information conveyed by the ears. People who sustain head injury are especially vulnerable to hearing loss or tinnitus, either temporary or permanent.

Pathophysiology

Sound travels to the brain: as follows: sound waves reach the outer ear and are conducted down the ear canal to the eardrum. The sound waves cause the eardrum to vibrate. These vibrations are passed through the 3 tiny ear bones in the middle ear, which transfer the vibrations to the fluid in the inner ear. The fluid moves hair cells, and the movement of the hair cells converts the vibrations into nerve impulses, which are then taken to the brain by the auditory nerve. The auditory nerve takes the impulses to the brainstem, which sends the impulses to the midbrain. Finally, the signal goes to the auditory cortex of the temporal lobe to be interpreted as sound.

Hearing loss is most commonly caused by long-term exposure to loud noises, from recreation or from work, that damage the hair cells, which do not grow back on their own.

Older people may lose their hearing from long exposure to noise, changes in the inner ear, changes in the middle ear, or from changes along the nerves from the ear to the brain.

Diagnosis

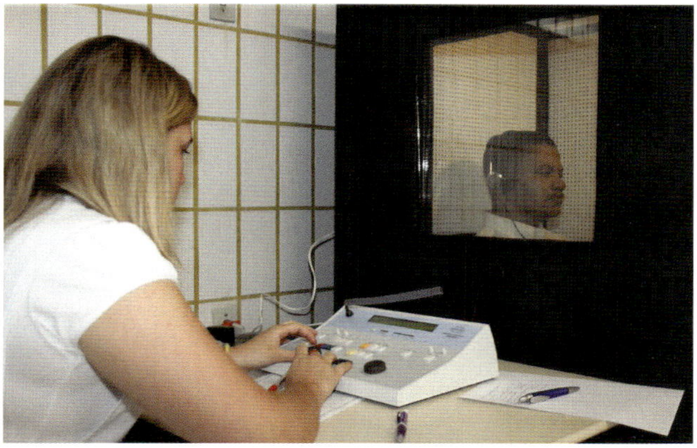

An audiologist conducting an audiometric hearing test in a sound-proof testing booth

Identification of a hearing loss is usually conducted by a general practitioner medical doctor, otolaryngologist, certified and licensed audiologist, school or industrial audiometrist, or other audiology technician. Diagnosis of the cause of a hearing loss is carried out by a specialist physician (audiovestibular physician) or otorhinolaryngologist.

Case History

A case history (usually a written form, with questionnaire) can provide valuable information about the context of the hearing loss, and indicate what kind of diagnostic procedures to employ. Case history will include such items as:

- major concern
- birth and pregnancy information
- medical history
- development history
- family history

- workplace environment
- home environment

Examination

- otoscopy, visual examination of the outer ear, ear canal, eardrum, and middle ear (through the translucent eardrum) using an optical instrument inserted into the ear canal called an otoscope
- tympanometry
- differential testing – the Weber, Rinne, Bing and Schwabach tests are simple manual tests of auditory function conducted with a low frequency (usually 512 Hz) tuning fork that can provide a quick indication of type of hearing loss: unilateral/bilateral, conductive, or other

Laboratory Testing

In case of infection or inflammation, blood or other body fluids may be submitted for laboratory analysis.

Hearing Tests

Hearing loss is generally measured by playing generated or recorded sounds, and determining whether the person can hear them. Hearing sensitivity varies according to the frequency of sounds. To take this into account, hearing sensitivity can be measured for a range of frequencies and plotted on an audiogram.

Another method for quantifying hearing loss is a speech-in-noise test. As the name implies, a speech-in-noise test gives an indication of how well one can understand speech in a noisy environment. A person with a hearing loss will often be less able to understand speech, especially in noisy conditions. This is especially true for people who have a sensorineural loss – which is by far the most common type of hearing loss. As such, speech-in-noise tests can provide valuable information about a person's hearing ability, and can be used to detect the presence of a sensorineural hearing loss. A recently developed digit-triple speech-in-noise test may be a more efficient screening test.

Otoacoustic emissions test is an objective hearing test that may be administered to toddlers and children too young to cooperate in a conventional hearing test. The test is also useful in older children and adults.

Auditory brainstem response testing is an electrophysiological test used to test for hearing deficits caused by pathology within the ear, the cochlear nerve and also within the brainstem. This test can be used to identify delay in the conduction of neural impulses due to tumours or inflammation but can also be an objective test of hearing thresholds. Other electrophysiological tests, such as cortical evoked responses, can look at the hearing pathway up to the level of the auditory cortex.

Scans

MRI and CT scans can be useful to identify the pathology of many causes of hearing loss. They are only needed in selected cases.

Classification

Hearing loss is categorized by type, severity, and configuration. Furthermore, a hearing loss may exist in only one ear (unilateral) or in both ears (bilateral). Hearing loss can be temporary or permanent, sudden or progressive.

Severity

The severity of a hearing loss is ranked according to ranges of nominal thresholds in which a sound must be so it can be detected by an individual. It is measured in decibels of hearing loss, or dB HL. The measurement of hearing loss in an individual is conducted over several frequencies, mostly 500 Hz, 1000 Hz, 2000 Hz and 4000 Hz. The hearing loss of the individual is the average of the hearing loss values over the different frequencies. Hearing loss can be ranked differently according to different organisations; and so, in different countries different systems are in use.

Hearing loss may be ranked as slight, mild, moderate, moderately severe, severe or profound as defined below:

- Slight: between 16 and 25 dB HL
- Mild:
    - for adults: between 26 and 40 dB HL
    - for children: between 20 and 40 dB HL
- Moderate: between 41 and 54 dB HL
- Moderately severe: between 55 and 70 dB HL
- Severe: between 71 and 90 dB HL
- Profound: 91 dB HL or greater
- Totally deaf: Have no hearing at all. This is called *anacusis*.

The 'Audiometric Classifications of Hearing Impairment' according to the International Bureau Audiophonology (BIAP) in Belgium is as follows:

- Normal or subnormal hearing: average tone loss is below 20 dB HL

- Mild hearing loss: average tone loss between 21 and 40 dB HL
- Moderate hearing loss
  - First degree: average tone loss between 41 and 55 dB HL
  - Second degree: average tone loss between 56 and 70 dB HL
- Severe hearing loss
  - First degree: average tone loss between 71 and 80 dB HL
  - Second degree: average tone loss between 81 and 90 dB HL
- Very severe hearing loss
  - First degree: average tone loss between 91 and 100 dB HL
  - Second degree: average tone loss between 101 and 110 dB HL
  - Third degree: average tone loss between 111 and 119 dB HL
- Total hearing loss or Cophosis: average tone loss is more than 120 dB HL

Hearing loss may affect one or both ears. If both ears are affected, then one ear may be more affected than the other. Thus it is possible, for example, to have normal hearing in one ear and none at all in the other, or to have mild hearing loss in one ear and moderate hearing loss in the other.

For certain legal purposes such as insurance claims, hearing loss is described in terms of percentages. Given that hearing loss can vary by frequency and that audiograms are plotted with a logarithmic scale, the idea of a percentage of hearing loss is somewhat arbitrary, but where decibels of loss are converted via a legally recognized formula, it is possible to calculate a standardized "percentage of hearing loss", which is suitable for legal purposes only.

Type

There are four main types of hearing loss, conductive hearing loss, sensorineural hearing loss, central deafness and combinations of conductive and sensorineural hearing losses which is called mixed hearing loss. An additional problem which is increasingly recognised is auditory processing disorder which is not a hearing loss as such but a difficulty perceiving sound.

- Conductive hearing loss

Conductive hearing loss is present when the sound is not reaching the inner ear, the cochlea. This can be due to external ear canal malformation, dysfunction of the eardrum or malfunction of the bones of the middle ear. The ear drum may show defects from small to total resulting in hearing loss of different degree. Scar tissue after ear infections may also make the ear drum dysfunction as well as when it is retracted and adherent to the medial part of the middle ear.

Dysfunction of the three small bones of the middle ear – malleus, incus, and stapes – may cause conductive hearing loss. The mobility of the ossicles may be impaired for different reasons and disruption of the ossicular chain due to trauma, infection or ankylosis may also cause hearing loss.

- Sensorineural hearing loss

Sensorineural hearing loss is one caused by dysfunction of the inner ear, the cochlea or the nerve that transmits the impulses from the cochlea to the hearing centre in the brain. The most common reason for sensorineural hearing loss is damage to the hair cells in the cochlea. Depending on the definition it could be estimated that more than 50% of the population over the age of 70 has impaired hearing.

- Central deafness

Damage to the brain can lead to a central deafness. The peripheral ear and the auditory nerve may function well but the central connections are damaged by tumour, trauma or other disease and the patient is unable to hear.

- Mixed hearing loss

Mixed hearing loss is a combination of conductive and sensorineural hearing loss. Chronic ear infection (a fairly common diagnosis) can cause a defective ear drum or middle-ear ossicle damages, or both. In addition to the conductive loss, a sensory component may be present.

- Central auditory processing disorder

This is not an actual hearing loss but gives rise to significant difficulties in hearing. One kind of auditory processing disorder is King-Kopetzky syndrome, which is characterized by an inability to process out background noise in noisy environments despite normal performance on traditional hearing tests.

Configuration

The shape of an audiogram shows the relative configuration of the hearing loss, such as a Carhart notch for otosclerosis, 'noise' notch for noise-induced damage, high frequency rolloff for presbycusis, or a flat audiogram for conductive hearing loss. In conjunction with speech audiometry, it may indicate central auditory processing disorder, or the presence of a schwannoma or other tumor. There are four general configurations of hearing loss:

1. Flat: thresholds essentially equal across test frequencies.

2. Sloping: lower (better) thresholds in low-frequency regions and higher (poorer) thresholds in high-frequency regions.
3. Rising: higher (poorer) thresholds in low-frequency regions and lower (better) thresholds in higher-frequency regions.
4. Trough-shaped ("cookie-bite" or "U" shaped): greatest hearing loss in the mid-frequency range, with lower (better) thresholds in low- and high-frequency regions.

Unilateral and Bilateral

People with unilateral hearing loss or single-sided deafness (SSD) have difficulty in:

- hearing conversation on their impaired side
- localizing sound
- understanding speech in the presence of background noise.

In quiet conditions, speech discrimination is approximately the same for normal hearing and those with unilateral deafness; however, in noisy environments speech discrimination varies individually and ranges from mild to severe.

One reason for the hearing problems these patients often experience is due to the head shadow effect. Newborn children with no hearing on one side but one normal ear could still have problems. Speech development could be delayed and difficulties to concentrate in school are common. More children with unilateral hearing loss have to repeat classes than their peers. Taking part in social activities could be a problem. Early aiding is therefore of utmost importance.

Prevention

It is estimated that half of cases of hearing loss are preventable. About 60% of hearing loss in children under the age of 15 can be avoided. A number of preventative strategies are effective including: immunization against rubella to prevent congenital rubella syndrome, immunization against *H. influenza* and *S. pneumoniae* to reduce cases of meningitis, and avoiding or protecting against excessive noise exposure. The World Health Organization also recommends immunization against measles, mumps, and meningitis, efforts to prevent premature birth, and avoidance of certain medication as prevention.

Noise exposure is the most significant risk factor for noise-induced hearing loss that can be prevented. Different programs exist for specific populations such as school-age children, adolescents and workers. Education regarding noise exposure increases the use of hearing protectors. The use of antioxidants is being studied for the prevention of noise-induced hearing loss, particularly for scenarios in which noise exposure cannot be reduced, such as during military operations.

Workplace Noise Regulation

Noise is widely recognized as an occupational hazard. In the United States, the National Institute for Occupational Safety and Health (NIOSH) and the Occupational Safety and Health Administration (OSHA) work together to provide standards and enforcement on workplace noise levels. The hierarchy of hazard controls demonstrates the different levels of controls to reduce or eliminate exposure to noise and prevent hearing loss, including engineering controls and personal protective equipment (PPE). Other programs and initiative have been created to prevent hearing loss in the workplace. For example, the Safe-in-Sound Award was created to recognize organizations that can demonstrate results of successful noise control and other interventions. Additionally, the Buy Quiet program was created to encourage employers to purchase quieter machinery and tools. By purchasing less noisy power tools like those found on the NIOSH Power Tools Database and limiting exposure to ototoxic chemicals, great strides can be made in preventing hearing loss.

Companies can also provide personal hearing protector devices tailored to both the worker and type of employment. Some hearing protectors universally block out all noise, and some allow for certain noises to be heard. Workers are more likely to wear hearing protector devices when they are properly fitted.

Often interventions to prevent noise-induced hearing loss have many components. A 2017 Cochrane review found that stricter legislation might reduce noise levels. Providing workers with information on their noise exposure levels was not shown to decrease exposure to noise. Ear protection, if used correctly, can reduce noise to safer levels, but often, providing them is not sufficient to prevent hearing loss. Engineering noise out and other solutions such as proper maintenance of equipment can lead to noise reduction, but further field studies on resulting noise exposures following such interventions are needed. Other possible solutions include improved enforcement of existing legislation and better implementation of well-designed prevention programmes, which have not yet been proven conclusively to be effective. The conclusion of the Cochrane Review was that further research could modify what is now regarding the effectiveness of the evaluated interventions.

Screening

The United States Preventive Services Task Force recommends screening for all newborns.

The American Academy of Pediatrics advises that children should have their hearing tested several times throughout their schooling:

- When they enter school
- At ages 6, 8, and 10

- At least once during middle school
- At least once during high school

While the American College of Physicians indicated that there is not enough evidence to determine the utility of screening in adults over 50 years old who do not have any symptoms, the American Language, Speech Pathology and Hearing Association recommends that adults should be screened at least every decade through age 50 and at 3-year intervals thereafter, to minimize the detrimental effects of the untreated condition on quality of life. For the same reason, the US Office of Disease Prevention and Health Promotion included as one of Healthy People 2020 objectives: to increase the proportion of persons who have had a hearing examination.

Treatment

Treatment depends on the specific cause if known as well as the extent, type and configuration of the hearing loss. Most hearing loss, that resulting from age and noise, is progressive and irreversible, and there are currently no approved or recommended treatments; management is by hearing aid. A few specific kinds of hearing loss are amenable to surgical treatment. In other cases, treatment is addressed to underlying pathologies, but any hearing loss incurred may be permanent.

There are a number of devices that can improve hearing in those who are deaf or hard of hearing or allow people with these conditions to manage better in their lives.

Hearing Aids

Hearing aids are devices that work to improve the hearing and speech comprehension of those with hearing loss. They work by magnifying the sound vibrations in the ear so that one can understand what is being said around them. Hearing aids have been shown to have a large beneficial effect in helping adults with mild to moderate hearing loss take part in everyday situations, and a smaller beneficial effect in improving physical, social, emotional and mental well-being in these people. Some people feel as if they cannot live without one because they say it is the only thing that keeps them engaged with the public. Conversely, there are many people who choose not to wear their hearing aids for a multitude of reasons. Up to 40% of adults with hearing aids for hearing loss fail to use them, or do not use them to their full effect. There are a number of reasons for this, stemming from factors such as: the aid amplifying background noises instead of the sounds they intended to hear; issues with comfort, care, or maintenance of the device; aesthetic factors; financial factors; and personal preference for quietness.

There is little evidence that interventions to encourage the regular use of hearing aids, (e.g. improving the information given to people about how to use hearing aids), increase daily hours of hearing aid use, and there is currently no agreed set of outcome measures for assessing this type of intervention.

Assistive Devices

Many deaf and hard of hearing individuals use assistive devices in their daily lives:

- Individuals can communicate by telephone using telephone typewriters (TTY). Other common names are textphone, minicom and telecommunications device for the deaf (TDD). These devices look like typewriters or word processors and transmit typed text over regular telephone lines. This allows communication through visual messaging. TTYs can transmit messages to individuals who don't have TTY by using the National Relay service which is an operator that acts as a messenger to each caller. For mobile phones, software apps are available to provide TDD/textphone functionality on some carriers/models to provide 2-way communications.
- There are several new telecommunications relay service technologies including IP Relay and captioned telephone technologies. A deaf or hard of hearing person can communicate over the phone with a hearing person via a human translator. Phone captioning is a service in which a hearing person's speech is captioned by a third party, enabling a deaf or hard of hearing person to conduct a conversation with a hearing person over the phone. Wireless, Internet and mobile phone/SMS text messaging are beginning to take over the role of the TDD.
- Real-time text technologies, involving streaming text that is continuously transmitted as it is typed or otherwise composed. This allows conversational use of text. Software programs are now available that automatically generate a closed-captioning of conversations. Examples include discussions in conference rooms, teleconference calls, classroom lectures and religious services.
- Instant messaging software.
- Videophones and similar video technologies can be used for distance communication using sign language. Video conferencing technologies permit signed conversations as well as permitting a sign language–English interpreter to voice and sign conversations between a deaf or hard of hearing person and that person's hearing party, negating the use of a TTY device or computer keyboard.
- Video relay service and video remote interpreting (VRI) services also use a third-party telecommunication service to allow a deaf or hard-of-hearing person to communicate quickly and conveniently with a hearing person, through a sign language interpreter.
- Hearing dogs are a specific type of assistance dog specifically selected and trained to assist the deaf and hard of hearing by alerting their handler to important sounds, such as doorbells, smoke alarms, ringing telephones, or alarm clocks.
- The advent of the Internet's World Wide Web and closed captioning has given

the deaf and hard of hearing unprecedented access to information. Electronic mail and online chat have reduced the need for deaf and hard-of-hearing people to use a third-party Telecommunications Relay Service to communicate with the hearing and other deaf people.

- A person with hearing loss cannot always hear the phone or distinguish their own ringtone from another. A signaling transmitter can be attached to a phone that will cause a light or a vibration device to activate. Transmitters can also be used to activate visual cues to represent fire alarms.
- Individuals with hearing loss require phones with amplifiers that have a higher power of amplification when compared to a regular phone. The Hearing Aid Telephone Interconnect System is a hands free amplification system which allows people to amplify sound when using telephones, cell phones, computer and pay phones by way of the attachment of a portable unit.

Wireless Hearing Aids

A wireless device has two main components: a transmitter and a receiver. The transmitter broadcasts the captured sound, and the receiver detects the broadcast audio and enables the incoming audio stream to be connected to accommodations such as hearing aids or captioning systems.

Three types of wireless systems are commonly used: FM, audio induction loop, and InfraRed. Each system has advantages and benefits for particular uses. FM systems can be battery operated or plugged into an electrical outlet. FM system produce an analog audio signal, meaning they have extremely high fidelity. Many FM systems are very small in size, allowing them to be used in mobile situations. The audio induction loop permits the listener with hearing loss to be free of wearing a receiver provided that the listener has a hearing aid or cochlear implant processor with an accessory called a "telecoil". If the listener does not have a telecoil, then he or she must carry a receiver with an earpiece. As with FM systems, the infrared (IR) system also requires a receiver to be worn or carried by the listener. An advantage of IR wireless systems is that people in adjoining rooms cannot listen in on conversations, making it useful for situations where privacy and confidentiality are required. Another way to achieve confidentiality is to use a hardwired amplifier, which contains or is connected to a microphone and transmits no signal beyond the earpiece plugged directly into it.

Surgical

There is no treatment, surgical or otherwise, for hearing loss due to the most common causes (age, noise, and genetic defects). For a few specific conditions, surgical intervention can provide a remedy:

- Surgical correction of superior canal dehiscence.

- Myringotomy, surgical insertion of drainage ventilation tubes in the tympanic membrane. Such placement is usually temporary until the underlying pathology (infection or other inflammation) can be resolved.
- Radiotherapy or surgical excision of vestibular schwannoma or acoustic neuroma, though, in most cases, it is unlikely that hearing will be preserved.
- Stapedectomy and stapedotomy for otosclerosis - replacement or reshaping of the stapes bone of the middle ear can restore hearing in cases of conductive hearing loss.

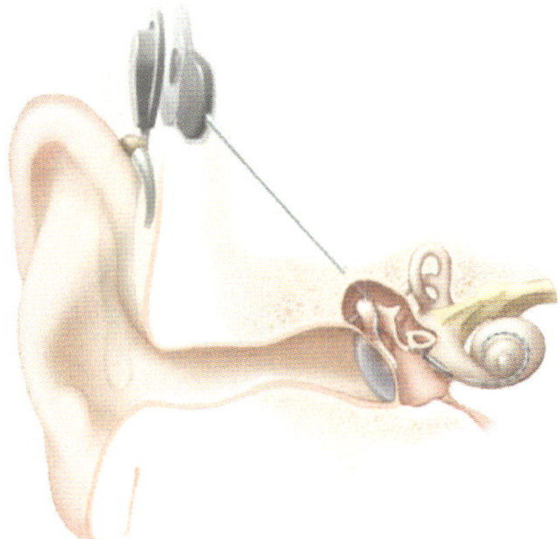

Illustration of a cochlear implant

Surgical and implantable hearing aids are an alternative to conventional external hearing aids. If the ear is dry and not infected, an air conduction aid could be tried; if the ear is draining, a direct bone condition hearing aid is often the best solution. If the conductive part of the hearing loss is more than 30–35 dB, an air conduction device could have problems overcoming this gap. A bone-anchored hearing aid could, in this situation, be a good option. The active bone conduction hearing implant Bonebridge is also an option. This implant is invisible under the intact skin and therefore minimises the risk of skin irritations.

Cochlear implants improve outcomes in people with hearing loss in either one or both ears. They work by artificial stimulation of the cochlear nerve by providing an electric impulse substitution for the firing of hair cells. They are expensive, and require programming along with extensive training for effectiveness.

Cochlear implants as well as bone conduction implants can help with single sided deafness. Middle ear implants or bone conduction implants can help with conductive hearing loss.

People with cochlear implants are at a higher risk for bacterial meningitis. Thus, meningitis vaccination is recommended. People who have hearing loss, especially those who develop a hearing problem in childhood or old age, may need support and technical adaptations as part of the rehabilitation process. Recent research shows variations in efficacy but some studies show that if implanted at a very young age, some profoundly impaired children can acquire effective hearing and speech, particularly if supported by appropriate rehabilitation.

Classroom

For a classroom setting, children with hearing loss often benefit from direct instruction and communication. One option for students is to attend a school for the Deaf, where they will have access to the language, communication, and education. Another option is to have the child attend a mainstream program, with special accommodation such as providing favorable seating for the child. Having the student sit as close to the teacher as possible improves the student's ability to hear the teacher's voice and to more easily read the teacher's lips. When lecturing, teachers can help the student by facing them and by limiting unnecessary noise in the classroom. In particular, the teacher can avoid talking when their back is turned to the classroom, such as while writing on a whiteboard.

Some other approaches for classroom accommodations include pairing deaf or hard of hearing students with hearing students. This allows the deaf or hard of hearing student to ask the hearing student questions about concepts that they have not understood. The use of CART (Communication Access Real Time) systems, where an individual types a captioning of what the teacher is saying, is also beneficial. The student views this captioning on their computer. Automated captioning systems are also becoming a popular option. In an automated system, software, instead of a person, is used to generate the captioning. Unlike CART systems, automated systems generally do not require an Internet connection and thus they can be used anywhere and anytime. Another advantage of automated systems over CART is that they are much lower in cost. However, automated systems are generally designed to only transcribe what the teacher is saying and to not transcribe what other students say. An automated system works best for situations where just the teacher is speaking, whereas a CART system will be preferred for situations where there is a lot of classroom discussion.

For those students who are completely deaf, one of the most common interventions is having the child communicate with others through an interpreter using sign language.

Sensorineural Hearing Loss

Having sensorineural hearing loss means you have damage to the hair cells in your inner ear or to the nerve pathways that lead from the inner ear to the brain. While much of sensorineural hearing loss is age-related, there are other factors that may cause it, too. Many people with sensorineural hearing loss report that they can hear, but they cannot understand speech. This is especially true in the presence of background noise, and it can be frustrating.

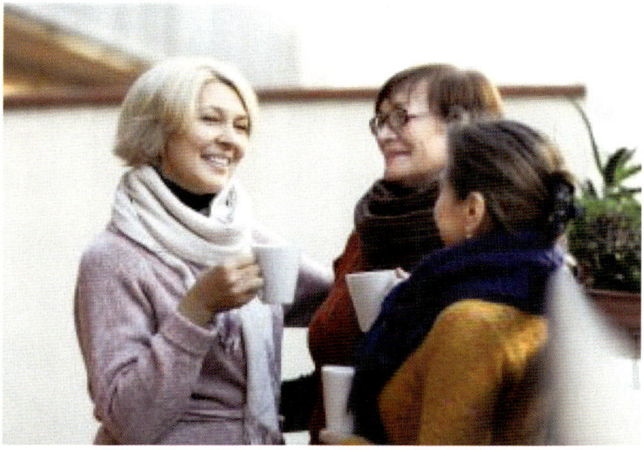

Sensorineural hearing loss can make communication a struggle.

There are two types of sensorineural hearing loss:

1. Congenital;
2. Acquired sensorineural hearing loss.

Congenital sensorineural hearing loss happens during pregnancy. Some causes include:

- Prematurity;
- Maternal diabetes;
- Lack of oxygen during birth;
- Genetics;
- Diseases passed from the mother to child in the womb, such as rubella.

Acquired sensorineural hearing loss occurs after birth. Causes can include:

- Aging: One of the most common conditions of growing older is presbycusis, or age-related hearing loss, affecting one in three Americans between the ages of 65-74. Because this type of loss occurs over time, typically in both ears, it's sometimes difficult to notice.
- Noise: According to the NIDCD, approximately 15 percent of Americans between the ages of 20 and 69 suffer from noise-induced hearing loss (NIHL). NIHL can be caused by exposure to a one-time loud noise, such as an explosion, or to sounds louder than 85 decibels (dB) over an extended period of time. If you have

to shout to be heard or your ears ring after attending a live concert or ballgame, your hearing health is at risk.

- Disease and infections: Viral infections, such as measles, meningitis and mumps can cause sensorineural hearing loss.
- Head or acoustic trauma: Damage to your inner ear can also be caused by a blow to the head or exposure to an extremely loud noise, such as an explosion. Many of our veterans suffer from sensorineural hearing loss due to time they spent around firearms, artillery and jet engines.
- Tumors: Examples of common tumors include acoustic neuroma, a benign tumor that affects the auditory system and cholesteatoma, an abnormal skin growth in the middle ear.
- Medications: According to the American Speech-Language-Hearing Association (ASHA), more than 200 medications and chemicals are ototoxic, or damaging to your hearing health. Some of those known to cause permanent damage include certain types of antibiotics, anti-inflammatory medications and cancer chemotherapy drugs like cisplatin and carboplatin.

Diagnosis

Case History

Before examination, a case history provides guidance about the context of the hearing loss.

- Major concern;
- Pregnancy and childbirth information;
- Medical history;
- Development history;
- Family history.

Otoscopy

Direct examination of the external canal and tympanic membrane (ear drum) with an otoscope, a medical device inserted into the ear canal that uses light to examine the condition of the external ear and tympanic membrane, and middle ear through the semi-translucent membrane.

Differential Testing

Differential testing is most useful when there is unilateral hearing loss, and distinguishes conductive from sensorineural loss. These are conducted with a low frequency tuning fork, usually 512 Hz, and contrast measures of air and bone conducted sound transmission.

- Weber test, in which a tuning fork is touched to the midline of the forehead, localizes to the normal ear in people with unilateral sensorineural hearing loss.
- Rinne test, which tests air conduction *vs.* bone conduction is positive, because both bone and air conduction are reduced equally.
- Less common Bing and Schwabach variants of the Rinne test.
- Absolute bone conduction (ABC) test.

Table. A table comparing sensorineural to conductive hearing loss

Criteria	*Sensorineural hearing loss*	*Conductive hearing loss*
Anatomical site	Inner ear, cranial nerve VIII, or central processing centers	Middle ear (ossicular chain), tympanic membrane, or external ear
Weber test	Sound localizes to normal ear in unilateral SNHL	Sound localizes to affected ear (ear with conductive loss) in unilateral cases
Rinne test	Positive Rinne; air conduction > bone conduction (both air and bone conduction are decreased equally, but the difference between them is unchanged).	Negative Rinne; bone conduction > air conduction (bone/air gap)

Other, more complex, tests of auditory function are required to distinguish the different types of hearing loss. Bone conduction thresholds can differentiate sensorineural hearing loss from conductive hearing loss. Other tests, such as oto-acoustic emissions, acoustic stapedial reflexes, speech audiometry and evoked response audiometry are needed to distinguish sensory, neural and auditory processing hearing impairments.

Tympanometry

A tympanogram is the result of a test with a tympanometer. It tests the function of the middle ear and mobility of the eardrum. It can help identify conductive hearing loss due to disease of the middle ear or eardrum from other kinds of hearing loss including SNHL.

Audiometry

An audiogram is the result of a hearing test. The most common type of hearing test is pure tone audiometry (PTA). It charts the thresholds of hearing sensitivity at a selection of standard frequencies between 250 and 8000 Hz. There is also high frequency pure tone audiometry which tests frequencies from 8000-20,000 Hz. PTA can be used to differentiate between conductive hearing loss, sensorineural hearing loss and mixed hearing loss. A hearing loss can be described by its degree i.e. mild, moderate, severe or profound, or by its shape i.e. high frequency or sloping, low frequency or rising, notched, U-shaped or 'cookie-bite', peaked or flat.

There are also other kinds of audiometry designed to test hearing acuity rather than sensitivity (speech audiometry), or to test auditory neural pathway transmission (evoked response audiometry).

Magnetic Resonance Imaging

MRI scans can be used to identify gross structural causes of hearing loss. They are used for congenital hearing loss when changes to the shape of the inner ear or nerve of hearing may help diagnosis of the cause of the hearing loss. They are also useful in cases where a tumour is suspected or to determine the degree of damage in a hearing loss caused by bacterial infection or auto-immune disease. Scanning is of no value in age-related deafness.

Pathophysiology

Sensory hearing loss is caused by abnormal structure or function of the hair cells of the organ of Corti in the cochlea. Neural hearing impairments are consequent upon damage to the eighth cranial nerve (the vestibulocochlear nerve) or the auditory tracts of the brainstem. If higher levels of the auditory tract are affected this is known as central deafness. Central deafness may present as sensorineural deafness but should be distinguishable from the history and audiological testing.

Cochlear Dead Regions in Sensory Hearing Loss

Hearing impairment may be associated with damage to the hair cells in the cochlea. Sometimes there may be complete loss of function of inner hair cells (IHCs) over a certain region of the cochlea; this is called a "dead region". The region can be defined in terms of the range of characteristic frequencies (CFs) of the IHCs and/or neurons immediately adjacent to the dead region.

Cochlear Hair Cells

Outer hair cells (OHCs) contribute to the structure of the Organ of Corti, which is situated between the basilar membrane and the tectorial membrane within the cochlea. The tunnel of corti, which runs through the Organ of Corti, divides the OHCs and the inner hair cells (IHCs). OHCs are connected to the reticular laminar and the Deiters' cells. There are roughly twelve thousand OHCs in each human ear, and these are arranged in up to five rows. Each OHC has small tufts of 'hairs', or cilia, on their upper surface known as stereocilia, and these are also arranged into rows which are graded in height. There are approximately 140 stereocilia on each OHC.

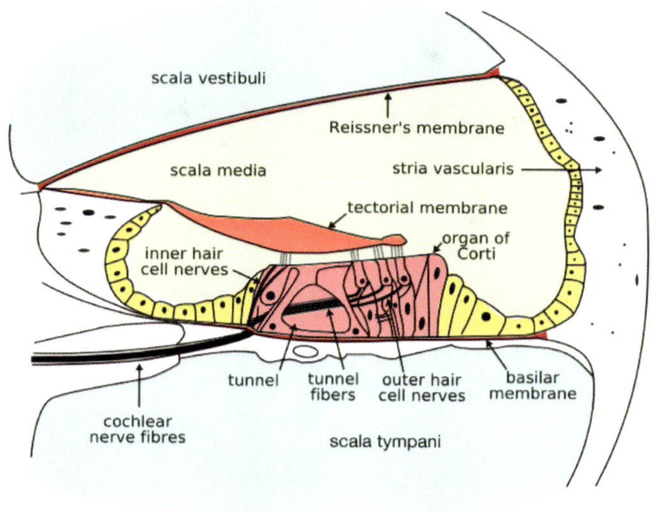

Figure: Cross-section of the cochlea.

The fundamental role of the OHCs and the IHCs is to function as sensory receptors. The main function of the IHCs is to transmit sound information via afferent neurons. They do this by transducing mechanical movements or signals into neural activity. When stimulated, the stereocilia on the IHCs move, causing a flow of electric current to pass through the hair cells. This electric current creates action potentials within the connected afferent neurons.

OHCs are different in that they actually contribute to the active mechanism of the cochlea. They do this by receiving mechanical signals or vibrations along the basilar membrane, and transducing them into electrochemical signals. The stereocilia found on OHCs are in contact with the tectorial membrane. Therefore, when the basilar membrane moves due to vibrations, the stereocilia bend. The direction in which they bend, dictates the firing rate of the auditory neurons connected to the OHCs.

The bending of the stereocilia towards the basal body of the OHC causes excitation of the hair cell. Thus, an increase in firing rate of the auditory neurons connected to the hair cell occurs. On the other hand, the bending of the stereocilia away from the basal body of the OHC causes inhibition of the hair cell. Thus, a decrease in firing rate of the auditory neurons connected to the hair cell occurs. OHCs are unique in that they are able to contract and expand (electromotility). Therefore, in response to the electrical stimulations provided by the efferent nerve supply, they can alter in length, shape and stiffness. These changes influence the response of the basilar membrane to sound. It is therefore clear that the OHCs play a major role in the active processes of the cochlea. The main function of the active mechanism is to finely tune the basilar membrane, and provide it with a high sensitivity to quiet sounds. The active mechanism is dependent on the cochlea being in good physiological condition. However, the cochlea is very susceptible to damage.

Hair Cell Damage

SNHL is most commonly caused by damage to the OHCs and the IHCs. There are two methods by which they might become damaged. Firstly, the entire hair cell might die. Secondly, the stereocilia might become distorted or destroyed. Damage to the cochlea can occur in several ways, for example by viral infection, exposure to ototoxic chemicals, and intense noise exposure. Damage to the OHCs results in either a less effective active mechanism, or it may not function at all. OHCs contribute to providing a high sensitivity to quiet sounds at a specific range of frequencies (approximately 2–4 kHz). Thus, damage to the OHCs results in the reduction of sensitivity of the basilar membrane to weak sounds. Amplification to these sounds is therefore required, in order for the basilar membrane to respond efficiently. IHCs are less susceptible to damage in comparison to the OHCs. However, if they become damaged, this will result in an overall loss of sensitivity.

Neural Tuning Curves

Frequency Selectivity

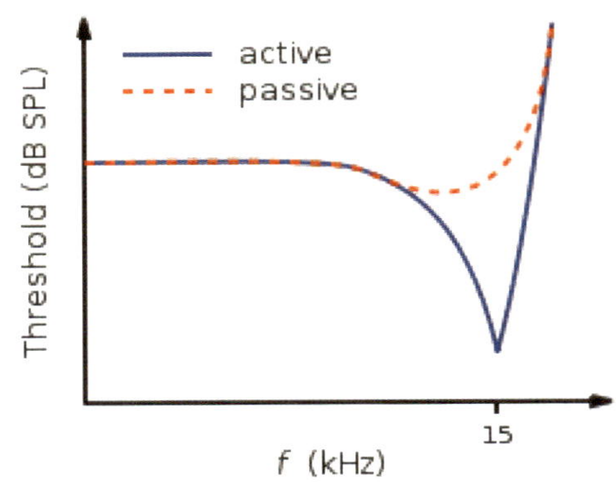

Figure: Neural tuning curve for normal hearing.

The traveling wave along the basilar membrane peaks at different places along it, depending on whether the sound is low or high frequency. Due to the mass and stiffness of the basilar membrane, low frequency waves peak in the apex, while high frequency sounds peak in the basal end of the cochlea. Therefore, each position along the basilar membrane is finely tuned to a particular frequency. These specifically tuned frequencies are referred to as characteristic frequencies (CF).

If a sound entering the ear is displaced from the characteristic frequency, then the strength of response from the basilar membrane will progressively lessen. The fine tuning of the basilar membrane is created by the input of two separate mechanisms. The first mechanism being a linear passive mechanism, which is dependent on the mechanical structure of the basilar membrane and its surrounding structures. The second mechanism is a non-linear active mechanism, which is primarily dependent on the functioning of the OHCs, and also the general physiological condition of the cochlea itself. The base and apex of the basilar membrane differ in stiffness and width, which cause the basilar membrane to respond to varying frequencies differently along its length. The base of the basilar membrane is narrow and stiff, resulting in it responding best to high frequency sounds. The apex of the basilar membrane is wider and much less stiff in comparison to the base, causing it to respond best to low frequencies.

This selectivity to certain frequencies can be illustrated by neural tuning curves. These demonstrate the frequencies a fiber responds to, by showing threshold levels (dB SPL) of auditory nerve fibers as a function of different frequencies. This demonstrates that auditory nerve fibers respond best, and hence have better thresholds at the fiber's characteristic frequency and frequencies immediately surrounding it. The basilar membrane is said to be 'sharply tuned' due to the sharp 'V' shaped curve, with its 'tip' centered at the auditory fibers characteristic frequency. This shape shows how few frequencies a fiber responds to. If it were a broader 'V' shape, it would be responding to more frequencies.

IHC vs OHC Hearing Loss

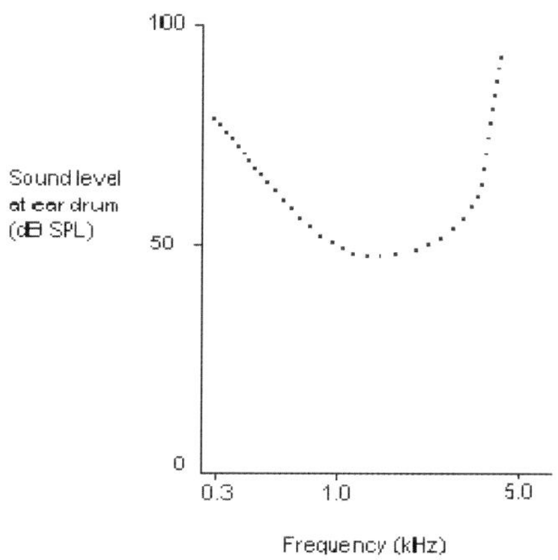

Figure: Neural tuning curve for OHC loss. Adapted from.

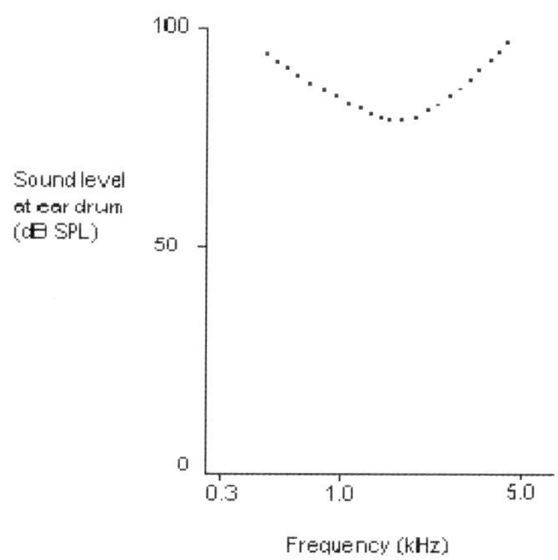

Figure: Neural tuning curve for OHC front row loss and IHC loss. Adapted from.

A normal neural tuning curve is characterised by a broadly tuned low frequency 'tail', with a finely tuned middle frequency 'tip'. However, where there is partial or complete damage to the OHCs, but with unharmed IHCs, the resulting tuning curve would show the elimination of sensitivity at the quiet sounds. I.e. where the neural tuning curve would normally be most sensitive (at the 'tip').

Where both the OHCs and the IHCs are damaged, the resulting neural tuning curve would show the elimination of sensitivity at the 'tip'. However, due to IHC damage, the whole tuning curve becomes raised, giving a loss of sensitivity across all frequencies. It is only necessary for the first row of OHCs to be damaged for the elimination of the finely tuned 'tip' to occur. This supports the idea that the incidence of OHC damage and thus a loss of sensitivity to quiet sounds, occurs more than IHC loss.

When the IHCs or part of the basilar membrane are damaged or destroyed, so that they no longer function as transducers, the result is a 'dead region'. Dead regions can be defined in terms of the characteristic frequencies of the IHC, related to the specific place along the basilar membrane where the dead region occurs. Assuming that there has been no shift in the characteristic frequencies relating to certain regions of the basilar membrane, due to the damage of OHCs. This often occurs with IHC damage. Dead regions can also be defined by the anatomical place of the non-functioning IHC (such as an "apical dead region"), or by the characteristic frequencies of the IHC adjacent to the dead region.

Dead Region Audiometry

Pure Tone Audiometry (PTA)

Dead regions affect audiometric results, but perhaps not in the way expected. For example, it may be expected that thresholds would not be obtained at the frequencies within the dead region, but would be obtained at frequencies adjacent to the dead region. Therefore, assuming normal hearing exists around the dead region, it would produce an audiogram that has a dramatically steep slope between the frequency where a threshold is obtained, and the frequency where a threshold cannot be obtained due to the dead region.

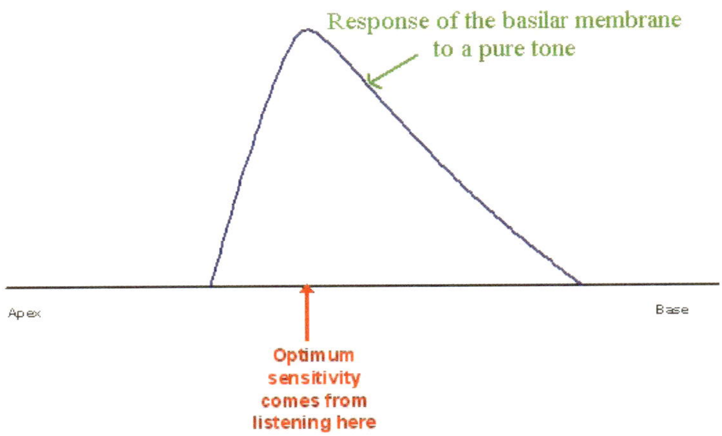

Figure: Response of the basilar membrane to a pure tone.

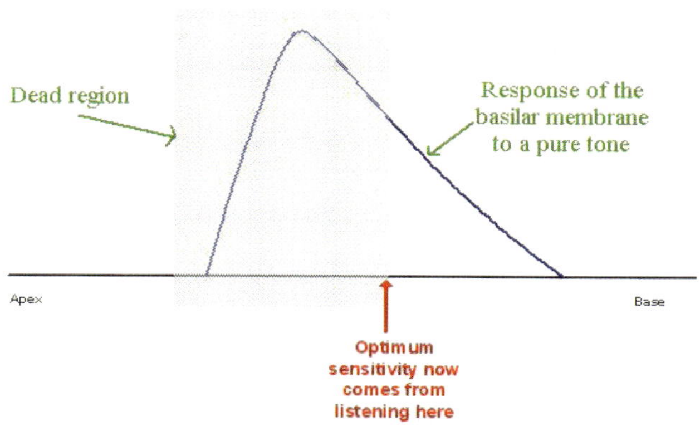

Figure: Response of the basilar membrane to a pure tone, when there is a dead region.

However, it appears that this is not the case. Dead regions cannot be clearly found via PTA audiograms. This may be because although the neurons innervating the dead region, cannot react to vibration at their characteristic frequency. If the basilar membrane vibration is large enough, neurons tuned to different characteristic frequencies such as those adjacent to the dead region, will be stimulated due to the spread of excitation. Therefore, a response from the patient at the test frequency will be obtained. This is referred to as "off-place listening", and is also known as 'off-frequency listening'. This will lead to a false threshold being found. Thus, it appears a person has better hearing than they actually do, resulting in a dead region being missed. Therefore, using PTA alone, it is impossible to identify the extent of a dead region.

Consequently, how much is an audiometric threshold affected by a tone with its frequency within a dead region? This depends on the location of the dead region. Thresholds at low frequency dead regions, are more inaccurate than those at higher frequency dead regions. This has been attributed to the fact that excitation due to vibration of the basilar membrane spreads upwards from the apical regions of the basilar membrane, more than excitation spreads downwards from higher frequency basal regions of the cochlea. This pattern of the spread of excitation is similar to the 'upward spread of masking' phenomenon. If the tone is sufficiently loud to produce enough excitation at the normally functioning area of the cochlea, so that it is above that areas threshold. The tone will be detected, due to off-frequency listening which results in a misleading threshold.

To help to overcome the issue of PTA producing inaccurate thresholds within dead regions, masking of the area beyond the dead region that is being stimulated can be used. This means that the threshold of the responding area is sufficiently raised, so that it cannot detect the spread of excitation from the tone. This technique has led to the suggestion that a low frequency dead region may be related to a loss of 40-50 dB. However, as one of the aims of PTA is to determine whether or not there is a dead region, it may be difficult to assess which frequencies to mask without the use of other tests.

Based on research it has been suggested that a low frequency dead region may produce a relatively flat loss, or a very gradually sloping loss towards the higher frequencies. As the dead region will be less detectable due to the upward spread of excitation. Whereas, there may be a more obvious steeply sloping loss at high frequencies for a high frequency dead region. Although it is likely that the slope represents the less pronounced downward spread of excitation, rather than accurate thresholds for those frequencies with non-functioning hair cells. Mid-frequency dead regions, with a small range, appear to have less effect on the patient's ability to hear in everyday life, and may produce a notch in the PTA thresholds. Although it is clear that PTA is not the best test to identify a dead region.

Psychoacoustic Tuning Curves (PTC) and Threshold Equalizing Noise (TEN) Tests

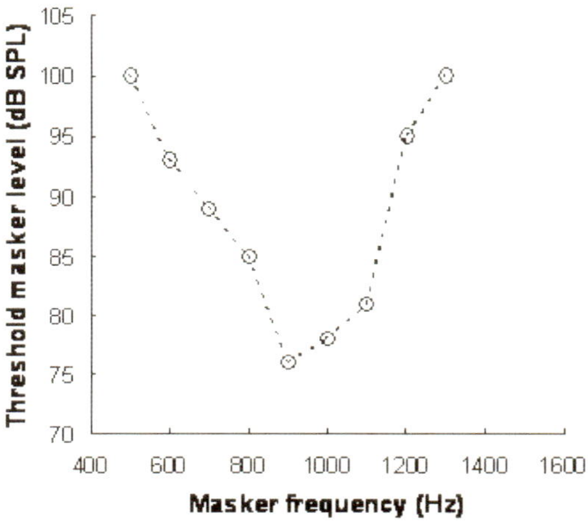

Figure: Psychoacoustical tuning curve.

Although some debate continues regarding the reliability of such tests, it has been suggested that psychoacoustic tuning curves (PTCs) and threshold-equalising noise (TEN) results may be useful in detecting dead regions, rather than PTA. PTCs are similar to neural tuning curves. They illustrate the level of a masker (dB SPL) tone at threshold, as a function of deviation from center frequency (Hz). They are measured by presenting a fixed low intensity pure tone while also presenting a narrow-band masker, with a varying center frequency. The masker level is varied, so that the level of masker needed to just mask the test signal is found for the masker at each center frequency. The tip of the PTC is where the masker level needed to just mask the test signal is the lowest. For normal hearing people this is when the masker center frequency is closest to the frequency of the test signal.

In the case of dead regions, when the test signal lies within the boundaries of a dead region, the tip of the PTC will be shifted to the edge of the dead region, to the area that is still functioning and detecting the spread of excitation from the signal. In the case of a low frequency dead region, the tip is shifted upwards indicating a low frequency dead region starting at the tip of the curve. For a high frequency dead region, the tip is shifted downwards from the signal frequency to the functioning area below the dead region. However, the traditional method of obtaining PTCs is not practical for clinical use, and it has been argued that TENs are not accurate enough. A fast method for finding PTCs has been developed and it may provide the solution. However, more research to validate this method is required, before it can be accepted clinically.

Perceptual Consequences of a Dead Region

Audiogram configurations are not good indicators of how a dead region will affect a person functionally, mainly due to individual differences. For example, a sloping audiogram is often present with a dead region, due to the spread of excitation. However, the individual may well be affected differently from someone with a corresponding sloped audiogram caused by partial damage to hair cells rather than a dead region. They will perceive sounds differently, yet the audiogram suggests that they have the same degree of loss. Huss and Moore investigated how hearing impaired patients perceive pure tones, and found that they perceive tones as noisy and distorted, more (on average) than a person without a hearing impairment. However, they also found that the perception of tones as being like noise, was not directly related to frequencies within the dead regions, and was therefore not an indicator of a dead region. This therefore suggests that audiograms, and their poor representation of dead regions, are inaccurate predictors of a patient's perception of pure tone quality.

Research by Kluk and Moore has shown that dead regions may also affect the patient's perception of frequencies beyond the dead regions. There is an enhancement in the ability to distinguish between tones that differ very slightly in frequency, in regions just beyond the dead regions compared to tones further away. An explanation for this may be that cortical re-mapping has occurred. Whereby, neurons which would normally be stimulated by the dead region, have been reassigned to respond to functioning areas near it. This leads to an over-representation of these areas, resulting in an increased perceptual sensitivity to small frequency differences in tones.

Vestibulocochlear Nerve Pathology

- Congenital deformity of the internal auditory canal,
- Neoplastic and pseudo-neoplastic lesions, with special detailed emphasis on schwannoma of the eighth cranial nerve (acoustic neuroma),
- Non-neoplastic Internal Auditory Canal/CerebelloPontine Angle pathology, including vascular loops.

Prevention

Presbycucis is the leading cause of SNHL and is progressive and nonpreventable, and at this time, we do not have either somatic or gene therapy to counter heredity-related

SNHL. But other causes of acquired SNHL are largely preventable, especially nosocusis type causes. This would involve avoiding environmental noise, and traumatic noise such as rock concerts and nightclubs with loud music. Use of noise attenuation measures like acoustic ear plugs is an alternative.

Treatment

Treatment modalities fall into three categories: pharmacological, surgical, and management. As SNHL is a physiologic degradation and considered permanent, there are as of this time, no approved or recommended treatments.

There have been significant advances in identification of human deafness genes and elucidation of their cellular mechanisms as well as their physiological function in mice. Nevertheless, pharmacological treatment options are very limited and clinically unproven. Such pharmaceutical treatments as are employed are palliative rather than curative, and addressed to the underlying cause if one can be identified, in order to avert progressive damage.

Profound or total hearing loss may be amenable to management by cochlear implants, which stimulate cochlear nerve endings directly. A cochlear implant is surgical implantation of a battery powered electronic medical device in the inner ear. Unlike hearing aids, which make sounds louder, cochlear implants do the work of damaged parts of the inner ear (cochlea) to provide sound signals to the brain. These consist of both internal implanted electrodes and magnets and external components. The quality of sound is different than natural hearing but may enable the recipient to better recognize speech and environmental sounds. Because of risk and expense, such surgery is reserved for cases of severe and disabling hearing impairment.

Management of sensorineural hearing loss involves employing strategies to support existing hearing such as lip-reading, enhanced communication etc. and amplification using hearing aids. Hearing aids are specifically tuned to the individual hearing loss to give maximum benefit.

Sudden Sensorineural Hearing Loss

Sudden sensorineural hearing loss (SSHL), commonly known as sudden deafness, occurs as an unexplained, rapid loss of hearing—usually in one ear—either at once or over several days. Nine out of ten people with SSHL lose hearing in only one ear. It should be considered a medical emergency. Delaying diagnosis and treatment may render treatment less effective or ineffective.

Experts estimate that SSHL strikes one person per 5,000 every year, typically adults in their 40s and 50s. The actual number of new cases of SSHL each year could be much higher because the condition often goes undiagnosed.

Presentation

Many people notice that they have SSHL when they wake up in the morning. Others first notice it when they try to use the deafened ear, such as when they use a phone. Still others notice a loud, alarming "pop" just before their hearing disappears. People with sudden deafness often become dizzy, have ringing in their ears (tinnitus), or both.

Diagnosis

SSHL is diagnosed via pure tone audiometry. If the test shows a loss of at least 30db in three adjacent frequencies, the hearing loss is diagnosed as SSHL. For example, a hearing loss of 30db would make conversational speech sound more like a whisper.

Causes

Only 10 to 15 percent of the cases diagnosed as SSHL have an identifiable cause. Most cases are classified as idiopathic, also called sudden idiopathic hearing loss (SIHL) and idiopathic sudden sensorineural hearing loss (ISSHL or ISSNHL) The majority of evidence points to some type of inflammation in the inner ear as the most common cause of SSNHL.

- Viral – The swelling may be due to a virus. A herpes type virus is believed to be the most common cause of sudden sensorineural hearing loss. The herpes virus lies dormant in our bodies and reactivates for an unknown reason;
- Vascular ischemia of the inner ear or cranial nerve VIII (CN8);
- Perilymph fistula, usually due to a rupture of the round or oval windows and the leakage of perilymph. The patient will usually also experience vertigo or imbalance. A history of trauma is usually present and changes to hearing or vertigo occur with alteration in intracranial pressure such as with straining; lifting, blowing etc;
- Autoimmune – can be due to an autoimmune illness such as systemic lupus erythematosus, granulomatosis with polyangiitis.

Treatment

About half of people with SSNHL will recover some or all of their hearing spontaneously, usually within one to two weeks from onset. Eighty-five percent of those who receive treatment from an otolaryngologist (sometimes called an ENT) will recover some of their hearing.

- Vitamins and antioxidants;
- Vasodilators;

- Betahistine (Betaserc), an anti-vertigo drug;
- Hyperbaric oxygen;
- Anti-inflammatory agents, primarily oral corticosteroids such as prednisone, methylprednisone;
- Intratympanic administration – Gel formulations are under investigation to provide more consistent drug delivery to the inner ear. Local drug delivery can be accomplished through intratympanic administration, a minimally invasive procedure where the ear drum is anesthetized and a drug is administered into the middle ear. From the middle ear, a drug can diffuse across the round window membrane into the inner ear. Intratympanic administration of steroids may be effective for sudden sensorineural hearing loss for some patients, but high quality clinical data has not been generated. Intratympanic administration of an anti-apoptotic peptide (JNK inhibitor) is currently being evaluated in late-stage clinical development.

Conductive Hearing Loss

A less common type of hearing loss is conductive hearing loss, which occurs when there is an obstruction or damage to the outer or middle ear that prevents sound from being conducted to the inner ear. Conductive hearing loss may be temporary or permanent, depending on the cause.

Causes

The causes of conductive hearing loss can be differentiated by which part of the ear they affect - either the outer or middle ear:

Outer ear

- Stenosis or a narrowing of the ear canal;
- Wax impaction;
- Exostoses (bone-like protrusions that can develop inside the ear canal and cause potential cause blockages);
- Otitis externa (also known as swimmer›s ear);
- Obstructions caused by foreign bodies inserted into the ear.

Middle ear

- A breach in the tympanic membrane caused by injury, ear infections or extreme and rapid air pressure changes;
- Tympanosclerosis or a thickening of the tympanic membrane;

- Otitis media or a buildup of fluid in the middle ear;
- Blockages in the Eustachian tube, which connects the middle ear to the back of the nose and throat;
- Otosclerosis, a rare medical condition that causes the middle ear bones to freeze up;
- Abnormal growths or tumors that form within the middle ear, such as cholesteatoma or glomus tumors;
- Ossicular chain discontinuity, or a break in the connection between the bones of the middle ear, caused by injury or heavy trauma.

Symptoms

Because the sensitive inner ear and auditory nerve are intact, an individual suffering from conductive hearing loss primarily has difficulty with the overall loudness of sounds, but not the clarity. Individuals with this kind of loss often find that turning up the volume of the radio or television is all it takes to improve their ability to hear. The following symptoms are also consistent with this type of loss:

- Easier time hearing out of one ear than the other;
- Pain in one or both ears;
- Sensation of pressure in one or both ears;
- Difficulty or frustration with telephone conversations;
- A foul odor coming from the ear canal;
- A feeling that one's own voice sounds louder or different.

Treatment

There are sometimes medical or surgical treatments that can improve the hearing ability for those with conductive hearing loss. For example, conductive losses caused by wax impaction, foreign objects, abnormal growths or ear infections can often be corrected with medical treatments, like extraction of earwax, antibiotics or surgical procedures. These causes usually result in temporary hearing losses. The treating physician and hearing healthcare professional will monitor hearing ability and work with the patient to determine when and if a hearing solution is needed.

Conductive hearing losses caused by other abnormalities, like stenosis of the ear canal, exostoses, otosclerosis and ossicular chain discontinuity are more difficult to treat medically and may be considered a permanent hearing loss. These conductive losses may be treated with traditional or bone-conduction hearing aids, bone-anchored implantable devices or middle ear implants. Assistive listening devices, like amplified telephones or headphones for television, may help provide a complete hearing solution.

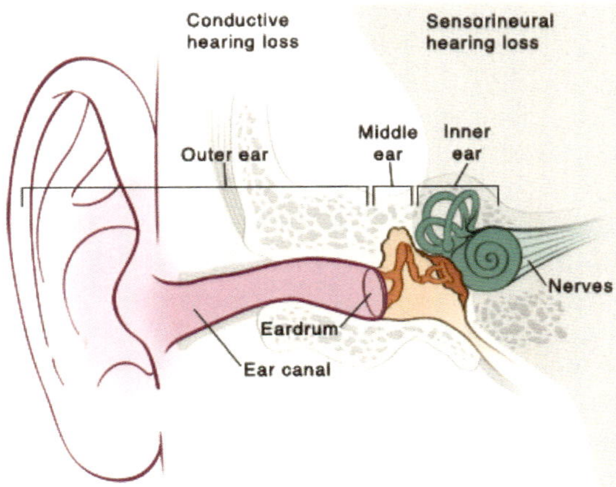

Nonsyndromic Deafness

Nonsyndromic hearing loss is a partial or total loss of hearing that is not associated with other signs and symptoms. In contrast, syndromic hearing loss occurs with signs and symptoms affecting other parts of the body.

Nonsyndromic hearing loss can be classified in several different ways. One common way is by the condition's pattern of inheritance: autosomal dominant (DFNA), autosomal recessive (DFNB), X-linked (DFNX), or mitochondrial (which does not have a special designation). Each of these types of hearing loss includes multiple subtypes. DFNA, DFNB, and DFNX subtypes are numbered in the order in which they were first described. For example, DFNA1 was the first type of autosomal dominant nonsyndromic hearing loss to be identified.

The characteristics of nonsyndromic hearing loss vary among the different types. Hearing loss can affect one ear (unilateral) or both ears (bilateral). Degrees of hearing loss range from mild (difficulty understanding soft speech) to profound (inability to hear even very loud noises). The term "deafness" is often used to describe severe-to-profound hearing loss. Hearing loss can be stable, or it may be progressive, becoming more severe as a person gets older. Particular types of nonsyndromic hearing loss show distinctive patterns of hearing loss. For example, the loss may be more pronounced at high, middle, or low tones.

Most forms of nonsyndromic hearing loss are described as sensorineural, which means they are associated with a permanent loss of hearing caused by damage to structures in the inner ear. The inner ear processes sound and sends the information to the brain in the form of electrical nerve impulses. Less commonly, nonsyndromic hearing loss is described as conductive, meaning it results from changes in the middle ear. The middle ear contains three tiny bones that help transfer sound from the eardrum to the inner ear. Some forms of nonsyndromic hearing loss, particularly a type called DFNX2, involve changes in both the inner ear and the middle ear. This combination is called mixed hearing loss.

Depending on the type, nonsyndromic hearing loss can become apparent at any time from infancy to old age. Hearing loss that is present before a child learns to speak is classified as prelingual or congenital. Hearing loss that occurs after the development of speech is classified as postlingual.

Between 2 and 3 per 1,000 children in the United States are born with detectable hearing loss in one or both ears. The prevalence of hearing loss increases with age; the condition affects 1 in 8 people in the United States age 12 and older, or about 30 million people. By age 85, more than half of all people experience hearing loss.

Causes

The causes of nonsyndromic hearing loss are complex. Researchers have identified more than 90 genes that, when altered, are associated with nonsyndromic hearing loss. Many of these genes are involved in the development and function of the inner ear. Mutations in these genes contribute to hearing loss by interfering with critical steps in processing sound. Different mutations in the same gene can be associated with different types of hearing loss, and some genes are associated with both syndromic and nonsyndromic forms. In many affected families, the factors contributing to hearing loss have not been identified.

Most cases of nonsyndromic hearing loss are inherited in an autosomal recessive pattern. About half of all severe-to-profound autosomal recessive nonsyndromic hearing loss results from mutations in the *GJB2* gene; these cases are designated DFNB1. The *GJB2* gene provides instructions for making a protein called connexin 26, which is a member of the connexin protein family. Mutations in another connexin gene, *GJB6*, can also cause DFNB1. The *GJB6* gene provides instructions for making a protein called connexin 30. Connexin proteins form channels called gap junctions, which allow communication between neighboring cells, including cells in the inner ear. Mutations in the *GJB2* or *GJB6* gene alter their respective connexin proteins, which changes the structure of gap junctions and may affect the function or survival of cells that are needed for hearing.

The most common cause of moderate autosomal recessive nonsyndromic hearing loss is mutations in the *STRC* gene. These mutations cause a form of the condition known as DFNB16. Mutations in more than 60 other genes can also cause autosomal recessive nonsyndromic hearing loss. Many of these gene mutations have been found in one or a few families.

Nonsyndromic hearing loss can also be inherited in an autosomal dominant pattern. Mutations in at least 30 genes have been identified in people with autosomal dominant nonsyndromic hearing loss; mutations in some of these genes (including *GJB2* and *GJB6*) can also cause autosomal recessive forms of the condition. Although no single gene is associated with a majority of autosomal dominant nonsyndromic hearing loss cases, mutations in a few genes, such as *KCNQ4* and *TECTA*, are relatively common. Mutations in many of the other genes associated with autosomal dominant nonsyndromic hearing loss have been found in only one or a few families.

X-linked and mitochondrial forms of nonsyndromic hearing loss are rare. About half of all X-linked cases are caused by mutations in the *POU3F4* gene. This form of the condition is designated DFNX2. Mutations in at least three other genes have also been identified in people with X-linked nonsyndromic hearing loss.

Mitochondrial forms of hearing loss result from changes in mitochondrial DNA (mtDNA). Mitochondria are structures within cells that convert the energy from food into a form that cells can use. Although most DNA is packaged in chromosomes within the nucleus, mitochondria also have a small amount of their own DNA. Only a few mutations in mtDNA have been associated with hearing loss, and their role in the condition is still being studied.

Mutations in some of the genes associated with nonsyndromic hearing loss can also cause syndromic forms of hearing loss, such as Usher syndrome (*CDH23* and *MYO7A*, among others), Pendred syndrome (*SLC26A4*), Wolfram syndrome (*WFS1*), and Stickler syndrome (*COL11A2*). It is often unclear how mutations in the same gene can cause isolated hearing loss in some individuals and hearing loss with additional signs and symptoms in others.

In addition to genetic changes, hearing loss can result from environmental factors or a combination of genetic risk and a person's environmental exposures. Environmental causes of hearing loss include certain medications, specific infections before or after birth, and exposure to loud noise over an extended period. Age is also a major risk factor for hearing loss. Age-related hearing loss (presbycusis) is thought to have both genetic and environmental influences.

Inheritance Pattern

As discussed above, nonsyndromic hearing loss has different patterns of inheritance. Between 75 and 80 percent of cases are inherited in an autosomal recessive pattern, which means both copies of the gene in each cell have mutations. Usually, each parent of an individual with autosomal recessive hearing loss carries one copy of the mutated gene but does not have hearing loss.

Another 20 to 25 percent of nonsyndromic hearing loss has an autosomal dominant pattern of inheritance, which means one copy of the altered gene in each cell is sufficient to cause the condition. Most people with autosomal dominant hearing loss inherit an altered copy of the gene from a parent who also has hearing loss.

Between 1 and 2 percent of cases have an X-linked pattern of inheritance. A condition is considered X-linked if the mutated gene that causes the disorder is located on the X chromosome, one of the two sex chromosomes in each cell. Males with X-linked nonsyndromic hearing loss tend to develop more severe hearing loss earlier in life than females who inherit a copy of the same gene mutation. A characteristic of X-linked inheritance is that fathers cannot pass X-linked traits to their sons.

Mitochondrial forms of the condition, which result from changes to mtDNA, account for less than 1 percent of all nonsyndromic hearing loss in the United States. These cases are inherited in a mitochondrial pattern, which is also known as maternal inheritance. This pattern of inheritance applies to genes contained in mtDNA. Because egg cells, but not sperm cells, contribute mitochondria to the developing embryo, children can only inherit disorders resulting from mtDNA mutations from their mother. These disorders can appear in every generation of a family and can affect both males and females, but fathers do not pass traits associated with changes in mtDNA to their children.

In some cases, hearing loss occurs in people with no history of the condition in their family. These cases are described as sporadic, and the cause of the hearing loss is often unknown. When hearing loss results from environmental factors, it is not inherited.

Evaluations Following Initial Diagnosis

To establish the extent of involvement and needs in an individual diagnosed with nonsyndromic hearing loss and deafness caused by biallelic pathogenic variants in *GJB2* (DFNB1), the following evaluations are recommended:

- Complete assessment of auditory acuity using age-appropriate tests such as ABR testing, auditory steady-state response (ASSR) testing, and pure tone audiometry;
- Ophthalmologic evaluation for refractive errors;
- Consultation with a clinical geneticist and genetic counselor.

Treatment of Manifestations

The following are indicated:

- Fitting with appropriate hearing aids;
- Enrollment in an appropriate educational program for the hearing impaired;
- Consideration of cochlear implantation (CI), an excellent habilitation option for persons with profound deafness;
- Recognition that, unlike with many clinical conditions, the management and treatment of severe-to-profound congenital deafness falls largely within the

purview of the social welfare and educational systems rather than the medical care system.

Surveillance

The following are appropriate:

- Annual examination by a physician familiar with hereditary hearing impairment;
- Repeat audiometry to confirm stability of hearing loss.

Agents/Circumstances to Avoid

Individuals with hearing loss should avoid environmental exposures known to cause hearing loss. Most important among these for persons with DFNB1 and mild-to-moderate hearing loss is avoidance of repeated overexposure to loud noises.

Evaluation of Relatives at Risk

If both *GJB2* pathogenic variants have been identified in the proband, it is appropriate to clarify the genetic status of at-risk sibs shortly after birth so that appropriate early support and management can be provided to the child and family.

Unilateral Hearing Loss

Unilateral hearing loss (UHL) means that hearing is normal in one ear but there is hearing loss in the other ear. The hearing loss can range from mild to very severe. UHL can occur in both adults and children.

Approximately 1 out of every 1,000 children is born with UHL, and nearly 3% of school-age children have UHL. Children with UHL are at higher risk for having academic, speech-language, and social-emotional difficulties than their normal hearing peers. This may be because UHL is often not identified, and the children do not receive intervention.

Your child may have had a hearing screening after he was born. It may have shown a hearing loss in only one ear. Or, the hearing loss may happen when he is older. This type of hearing loss will not keep him from learning to talk. However, he may have some speech and language delays because of the UHL. We do not yet know why some children have problems and others do not.

Below are some possible causes of UHL:

- Hearing loss that runs in the family (genetic or hereditary);
- An outer, middle, or inner ear abnormality;

- Some syndromes;
- Illnesses or infections;
- Head injury;
- Exposure to loud noise;
- Traumatic brain injury (TBI).

Signs of UHL

It may be hard to see signs of UHL in babies and young children. A child with UHL may have:

- Trouble finding where sounds come from, called localization. It helps direct us to who is talking at any moment. Your child may miss some of a message if he does not know who is talking. It is also important for safety. If your child is near a street, he may have trouble knowing where a horn is coming from. This could put him in danger.
- Problems understanding speech in noisy places. It is easier to focus on sounds when you hear from both ears.
- Problems hearing you from another room or from outside. Sounds seem louder when we hear with both ears. When two normal-hearing ears hear together, sound seems louder. With UHL, your child may hear speech but not understand what is said.

When your child has trouble hearing, she may:

- Get upset at not being able to hear.
- Be very tired by the end of the day. This happens when she has to focus on speech all day.
- Seem like she is not paying attention.
- Answer questions wrong.
- "Act out" or have tantrums when frustrated.
- Turn the TV or radio on too loud.

Testing for UHL

Any child with hearing loss should be seen by an ear, nose, and throat doctor, or ENT. The ENT will look in your child's ears and check for fluid in the middle ear. The ENT may order special tests to find out why your child has UHL.

An audiologist can test your child's hearing. This will include tests of his middle ear. The audiologist may do special hearing tests, if needed.

Your child may see a speech-language pathologist, or SLP. The SLP will test her speech and language. The local early intervention, or EI, program can see children under 3 years old. Your child may get services from the EI program. They can suggest activities you can do at home to help your child.

Treatment for UHL

Your child may be able to use a hearing aid. It depends on his age and the amount of hearing loss. Your audiologist will help you decide what is best for your child.

Your child may need speech and language treatment. An SLP can help your child learn to speak clearly. The SLP can teach your child to listen to sounds and find where they come from. Both the audiologist and SLP can suggest ways to help your child hear at home and at school.

Tips for Helping Children with UHL

There are things you can do to help your child hear and learn. They include:

- Making sure that your child's "good" ear is facing sounds. Think about this when you are feeding your child and when you are in the car. Your child should face the person speaking.
- Look at your child when speaking to her.
- Talk about what you are doing. Say things like, "I am making a sandwich," or "It's time to wash the dishes." This teaches your child words and sentences.
- Repeat words. Use new words to help your child say more.
- Play listening games with your child. See who can hear the phone ring or who hears the dog bark.
- Get your child's attention before talking to him. This may help him focus on what you say.
- Help your child find where sounds come from.
- Make sure your child puts the phone to her good ear.
- Speak louder than usual, and face your child. Try not to talk to him from another room.
- Teach your child to take care of her hearing. Have her wear earplugs when she is around loud noises. Make sure she does not turn the volume up too loud when using headphones.

Tips for School

- Look closely at the setup when choosing a day care center or preschool. Try to avoid situations where many classes are within one large area. This will be noisy.
- Make sure that your child is seated near the teacher with her better ear facing the teacher. Being closer lets your child hear and see the teacher better.
- Ask that the teacher give your child pictures and handouts to go along with verbal lessons.
- Make sure that your child is not seated with his normal-hearing ear facing a noisy hallway or air conditioner.
- Make sure the teacher knows how your child's hearing aid or frequency modulation (FM) system works. Have extra batteries for these systems in the classroom.
- Talk to your child's teacher to monitor your child's progress. If you or the teacher have concerns, ask for further testing.
- Let your child's teacher know that your child may have trouble localizing sound. For example, she may not hear when someone calls her name on the playground.
- Seek help if you notice your child is becoming frustrated or having trouble making friends.
- Share with your child's teacher what you have learned about UHL, Give the teacher written information about UHL.
- Ask to talk with an educational audiologist or other professional who works with children who have hearing loss. This person can work with your child and the teacher on strategies to help your child in school and with friends. This person can also make sure that the classroom has the best acoustics. These are changes to the room that lower noise levels.

Tips for Home

- Make your home "listening friendly." There are things you can do to reduce noise. Use carpeting and cloth curtains. Replace buzzing fluorescent lights. Run noisy appliances, like the dishwasher or washing machine, when your child is not home or is sleeping.
- Try not to let your child's normal-hearing ear face noise sources, like the dishwasher, air conditioner, or radio.
- Do not have the TV or radio on while eating dinner or at other times when you are talking with your child.

- Be aware of where your child sits at the dinner table. Try to have the child facing those who will be talking to him.
- Be aware of where your child is seated in the car. For example, a child with hearing loss in her right ear should sit behind the passenger seat. This lets her normal-hearing ear face the other people in the car.
- Do not give your child instructions from another room. He will likely hear your voice but may not understand what you are saying.
- Teach others the things that you have learned about helping your child.
- Make sure that your child's hearing aid is working. A hearing aid that does not work is much worse than no hearing aid at all.

Spatial Hearing Loss

Spatial hearing is a central part of everyday listening. The ability to determine the direction of a sound source is a natural and effortless skill that is only remarked on in rare or challenging circumstances, such as when a driver cannot determine the direction of the siren of a passing ambulance. But spatial hearing performance by hearing-impaired listeners is considerably degraded, and generally hearing aids do not offer any benefit.

In most circumstances — excepting only if a sound source is *exactly* directly ahead, above, or behind — the fine details of a sound's waveform at the left ear will differ in some way from those at the right ear. The auditory system is sensitive to these interaural ("between the ears") differences. Imagine that the source is to the right of someone's head. The left ear is further from the source than the right ear, by about 18-20 cm, so the sound will arrive there a fraction of a millisecond after it arrives at the right ear. The left ear is also in the acoustic shadow cast by the head, so the sound's level will be less there than at the right ear. Both interaural cues physically occur at all frequencies, but their importance varies with frequency. The interaural level differences (ILDs) can reach 20 or 30 dB at frequencies around 5-10 kHz, but are less than 5 dB below 500 Hz. ILDs are therefore generally regarded as being most useful at high frequencies. Conversely, the interaural time differences (ITDs) — at most, about 600-800 millionths of a second — are primarily a low-frequency cue, useful up to around 1500 Hz.

Many laboratory experiments have demonstrated that normal-hearing listeners are remarkably sensitive to these two cues: at best, people can discriminate changes of about 0.5 dB of ILD or 10 millionths of a second of ITD. But in everyday listening people are never called onto discriminate pure changes in ILD or ITD in isolation: when the direction of a source changes, both cues vary. At best, the discrimination for changes in direction is about 1 degree of spatial angle. This is the "minimal audible angle": one can reliably distinguish the left *vs.* right direction of two sounds, presented in quiet, 1 degree apart. These measurements can be made directly using very closely-spaced loudspeakers or with robot arms to accurately move loudspeakers by very small amounts.

An alternative approach is to use a fixed loudspeaker array with relatively large spacing between loudspeakers, such as 15 degrees, and then measure how inaccurate listeners are at reporting the direction of sounds presented from them.

One degree of angle is really not very much: it corresponds to the apparent width of the index fingernail held at arm's length. Comparative measurements in mammals have demonstrated that humans have amongst the best performance: of all species measured so far; only dolphins and elephants do as well or better . It is curious why we should be so good at distinguishing sound direction in quiet. Perhaps it is a by-product — an evolutionary spandrel— of something else, such as better directional resolution for sounds in noise, or dealing with moving sounds, or even helping to guide visual attention.

The inability to distinguish spatial cues is known as spatial hearing loss. For example, if a person suffers from spatial loss of hearing, they would likely be unable to tell where a sound came from. They would also have a difficult time picking one person's voice out of a crowd. People with this condition find it hard to cut out background sounds in noisy areas, such as bars, restaurants, or movie theaters. Perhaps surprisingly, the ear is not the source of spatial hearing loss. Instead, it is thought to occur within the brain pathways that interpret noise.

Spatial loss of hearing is especially common in children as well as adults over the age of 60. However, it can occur in anyone, regardless of age. This can be especially frustrating for children in school – they find it hard to differentiate the teacher's voice from other noises in class.

Corpus Callosum

Many neuroscience studies have facilitated the development and refinement of a speech processing model. This model shows cooperation between the two hemispheres of the brain, with asymmetric inter-hemispheric and intrahemispheric connectivity consistent with the left hemisphere specialization for phonological processing. The right hemisphere is more specialized for sound localization, while auditory space representation in the brain requires the integration of information from both hemispheres.

The corpus callosum (CC) is the major route of communication between the two hemispheres. At maturity it is a large mass of white matter and consists of bundles of fibres linking the white matter of the two cerebral hemispheres. Its caudal and splenium portions contain fibres that originate from the primary and second auditory cortices, and from other auditory responsive areas. Transcallosal interhemispheric transfer of auditory information plays a significant role in spatial hearing functions that depend on binaural cues. Various studies have shown that despite normal audiograms, children with known auditory interhemispheric transfer deficits have particular difficulty localizing sound and understanding speech in noise.

The CC of the human brain is relatively slow to mature with its size continuing to increase until the fourth decade of life. From this point it then slowly begins to shrink. LiSN-S SRT scores show that the ability to understand speech in noisy environments develops with age, is beginning to be adult like by 18 years and starts to decline between 40 and 50 years of age.

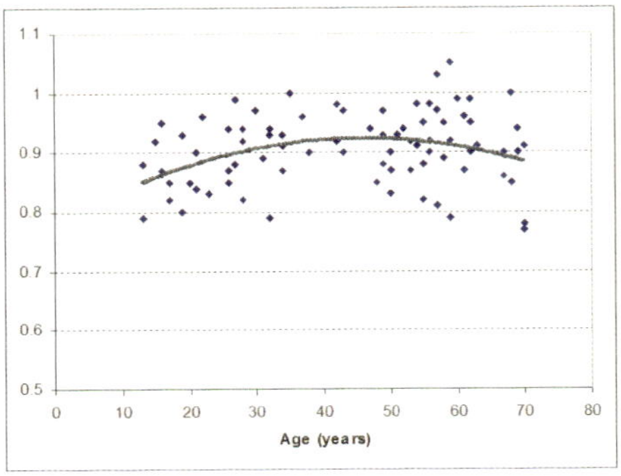

CC density (and myelination) increases during childhood, and into early adulthood, peaking and then decreasing during the fourth decade.

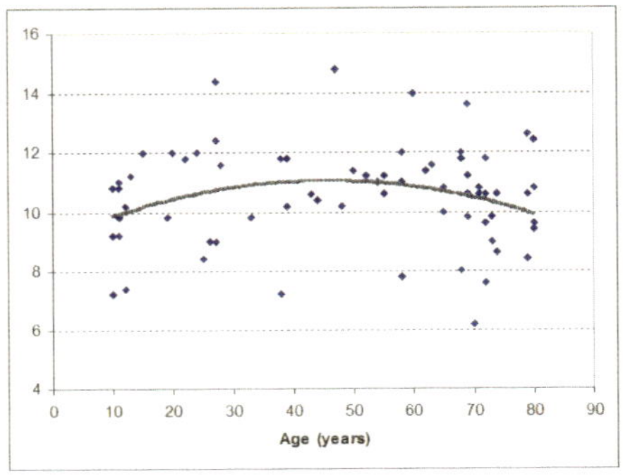

Spatial Hearing Advantage (dB) continues to increase through childhood and into adulthood. It then begins to decrease again during the fourth decade.

Roles of the SOC and the MOC

The medial olivocochlear bundle (MOC) is part of a collection of brainstem nuclei known as the superior olivary complex (SOC). The MOC innervates the outer hair cells of the cochlea and its activity is able to reduce basilar-membrane responses to sound by reducing the gain of cochlear amplification.

In a quiet environment when speech from a single talker is being listened to, then the MOC efferent pathways are essentially inactive. In this case the single speech stream enters both ears and its representation ascends the two auditory pathways. The stream arrives at both the right and left auditory cortices for eventual speech processing by the left hemisphere.

In a noisy environment the MOC efferent pathways are required to be active in two distinct ways. The first is an automatic response to the multiple sound streams arriving at the two ears, while the second is a top-down corticofugal attention driven response. The purpose of both is an attempt to enhance the signal to noise ratio between the speech stream being listened to and all other sound streams.

The automatic response involves the MOC efferents inhibiting the output of the cochlear of the left ear. The output of the right ear is therefore dominant and only the right hemispace streams (with their direct connection to the speech processing areas of the left hemisphere) travel up the auditory pathway. With children the underdeveloped

Corpus Callosum (CC) is unable, in any case, to transfer auditory streams arriving (from the left ear) at the right hemisphere to the left hemisphere.

With adults with a mature CC, an attention driven (conscious) decision to attend to one particular sound stream is the trigger for further MOC activity. The 3D spatial representation of the multiple streams of the noisy environment (a function of the right hemisphere) enables a choice of the ear to be attended to. As a consequence, instruction may be given to the MOC efferents to inhibit the output of the right cochlear rather than the left cochlear. If the speech stream being attended to is from the left hemispace it will arrive at the right hemisphere and access speech processing via the CC.

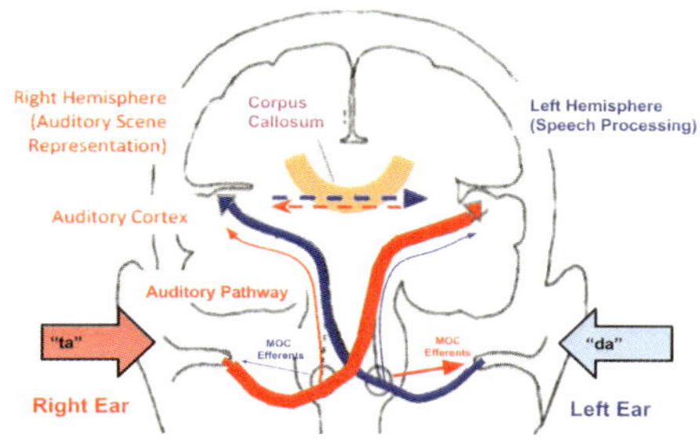

Noisy Environment: The MOC efferents automatic response is to inhibit the left ear cochlea thus favouring the sounds arriving at the right ear. This is the right ear advantage (REA).

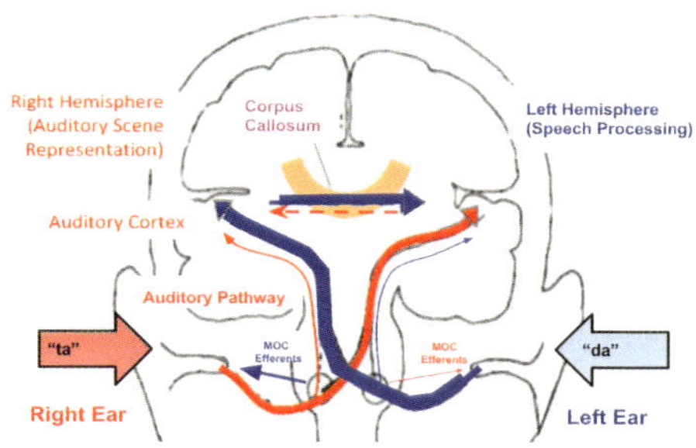

Noisy Environment: An attention driven optional response with the MOC efferents inhibiting the right ear cochlea. The sounds arriving at the left ear are favoured.

Diagnosis

Spatial hearing loss can be diagnosed using the Listening in Spatialized Noise – Sentences test (LiSN-S), which was designed to assess the ability of children with central auditory processing disorder (CAPD) to understand speech in background noise. The LiSN-S allows audiologists to measure how well a person uses spatial (and pitch information) to understand speech in noise. Inability to use spatial information has been found to be a leading cause of CAPD in children.

Test participants repeat a series of target sentences which are presented simultaneously with competing speech. The listener's speech reception threshold (SRT) for target sentences is calculated using an adaptive procedure. The targets are perceived as coming from in front of the listener whereas the distracters vary according to where they are perceived spatially (either directly in front or either side of the listener). The vocal identity of the distracters also varies (either the same as, or different from, the speaker of the target sentences).

Performance on the LISN-S is evaluated by comparing listeners' performances across four listening conditions, generating two SRT measures and three "advantage" measures. The advantage measures represent the benefit in dB gained when either talker, spatial, or both talker and spatial cues are available to the listener. The use of advantage measures minimizes the influence of higher order skills on test performance. This serves to control for the inevitable differences that exist between individuals in functions such as language or memory.

Dichotic listening tests can be used to measure the efficacy of the attentional control of cochlear inhibition and the inter-hemispheric transfer of auditory information. Dichotic listening performance typically increases (and the right-ear advantage decreases) with the development of the Corpus Callosum (CC), peaking before the fourth decade. During middle age and older the auditory system ages, the CC reduces in size, and dichotic listening becomes worse, primarily in the left ear. Dichotic listening tests typically involve two different auditory stimuli (usually speech) presented simultaneously, one to each ear, using a set of headphones. Participants are asked to attend to one or (in a divided-attention test) both of the messages.

The activity of the medial olivocochlear bundle (MOC) and its inhibition of cochlear gain can be measured using a Distortion Product Otoacoustic Emission (DPOE) recording method. This involves the contralateral presentation of broadband noise and the measurement of both DPOAE amplitudes and the latency of onset of DPOAE suppression. DPOAE suppression is significantly affected by age and becomes difficult to detect by approximately 50 years of age.

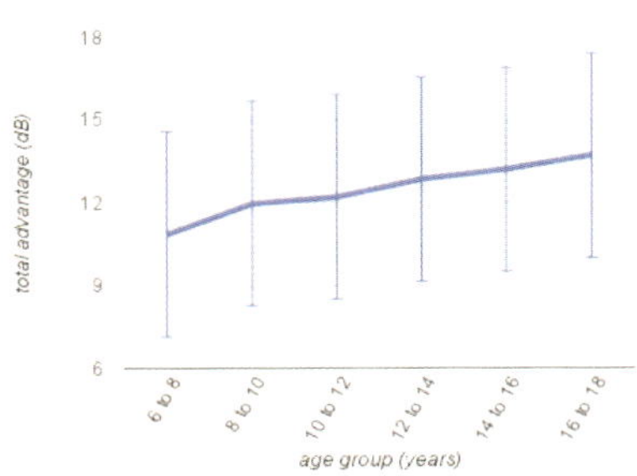

Spatial Hearing Advantage (dB) slowly increases through childhood and into adulthood.

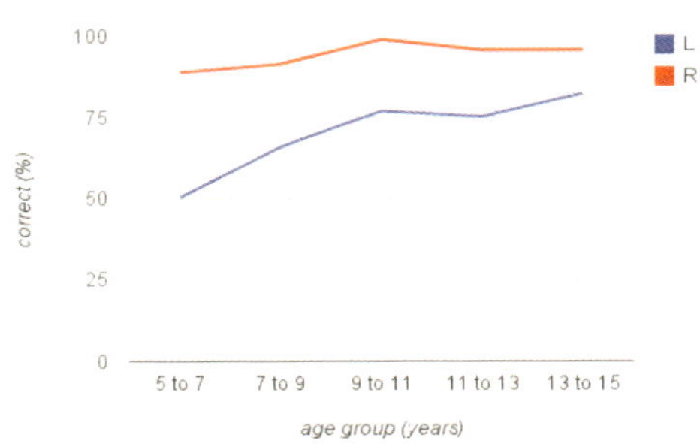

The left ear disadvantage slowly decreases through childhood and into adulthood. The right ear advantage still exists as children move into early adulthood.

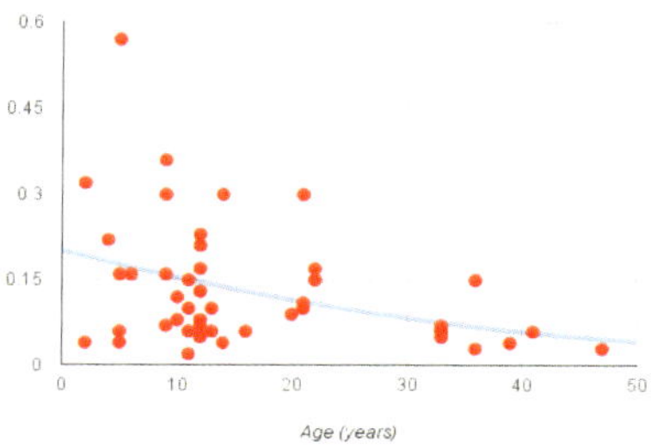

The amplitude of contralateral DPOAE suppression decreases with ageing.

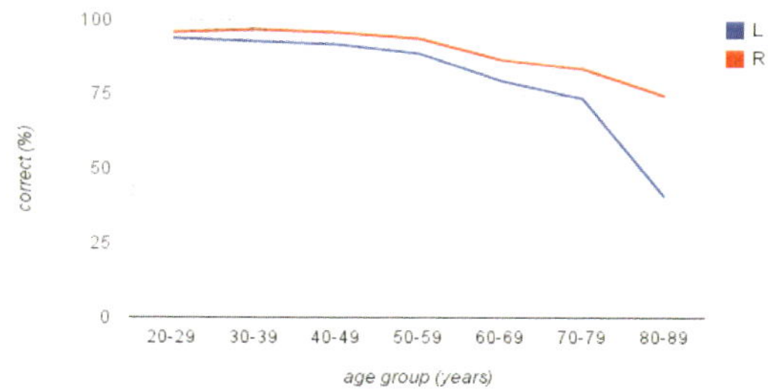

By early adulthood the left ear disadvantage is negligible. The right ear advantage re-establishes itself from middle to old age, primarily due to the faster falling of the left ear performance.

Occupational Hearing Loss

Noise is the insidious of all industrial pollutants, involving every industry and causing severe hearing loss in every country in the world. Exposure to excessive noise is the major avoidable cause of permanent hearing impairment. Worldwide, 16% of the disabling hearing loss in adults is attributed to occupational noise, ranging from 7 to 21% in the various subregions. The estimated cost of noise to developed countries ranges from 0.2 to 2% of the gross domestic product (GDP). Noise-induced hearing loss (NIHL) is bilateral and symmetrical, usually affecting the higher frequencies (3k, 4k or 6k Hz) and then spreading to the lower frequencies (0.5k, 1k or 2k Hz). Other major health effects are lack of concentration, irritation, fatigue, headache, sleep disturbances, etc. The major industries responsible for excessive noise and exposing workers to hazardous levels of noise are textile, printing, saw mills, mining, etc. Hearing protectors should be used when engineering controls and work practices are not feasible for reducing noise exposure to safe levels. Earmuffs, ear plugs and ear canal caps are the main types of hearing protectors. Awareness should be created among workers about the harmful effects of noise on hearing and other body systems by implementing compulsory education and training programs.

Occupational hearing loss includes acoustic traumatic injury and noise-induced hearing loss (NIHL), and can be defined as a partial or complete hearing loss in one or both ears as the result of ones employment. Exposure to excessive noise is the major avoidable cause of permanent hearing impairment worldwide. NIHL is an important public health priority because as populations live longer and industrialization spreads, NIHL will add substantially to the global burden of disability. In many countries, excessive noise is the biggest compensatable occupational hazard. Worldwide, 16% of the disabling hearing loss in adults is attributed to occupational noise, ranging from 7 to 21% in the various subregions. The estimated cost of noise to developed countries ranges from 0.2 to 2% of the GDP, where it is the cause of more than one-third of the hearing impairments. The effects of the exposure to occupational noise are higher in the developing regions.

Noise-induced Hearing Loss

NIHL is generally used to denote the cumulative, permanent loss of hearing that develops gradually after months or years of exposure to high levels of noise. It has long been recognized as a problem in occupations associated with prominent noise. NIHL is the second most common form of acquired hearing loss after age-related loss (presbycusis), with studies showing that people who are exposed to noise levels higher than 85 db suffered from NIHL. A typical NIHL is of a sensory neural type involving injury to the inner ear. It is bilateral and symmetrical, usually affecting the higher frequencies (3k, 4k or 6k Hz) and then spreading to the lower frequencies (0.5k, 1k or 2k Hz). Impairment of hearing at high frequencies will initially cause a loss of clarity in perceived speech and then interfere with daily activities as hearing loss progresses. Hearing loss-related symptoms, such as trouble in normal and telephone conversation, turning up the radio/television volume and tinnitus, usually occur in the early stages of NIHL. Other major health effects due to the noise pollution are lack of concentration, irritation, fatigue, headache, sleep disturbances, etc. The risk of hearing loss and injury to the ears increases with the sound intensity, the length of time an employee is exposed to noise and the individual susceptibility to NIHL.

Pathogenesis of Noise-Induced Hearing Loss

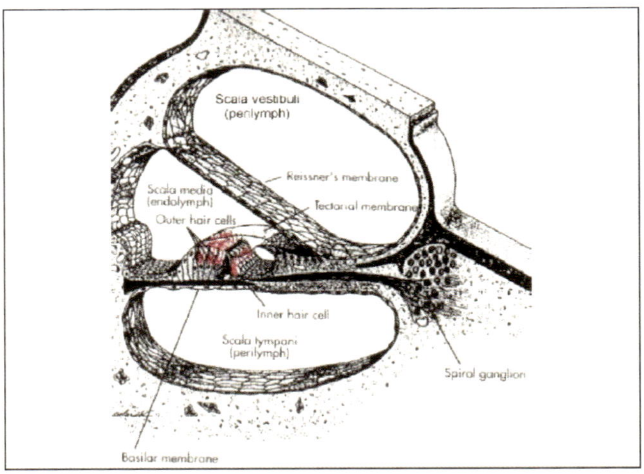

A cross section of the human cochlea

Sound travels from external ear and falls on the tympanic membrane, which is then set into vibration and these vibrations are transmitted to the middle ear where the sensory hair cells in the cochlea are responsible for initiating the neural impulses that carry information to the brain regarding the sounds. The human cochlea has one row of inner hair cells and three rows of outer hair cells. The outer rows of hair cells run throughout the length of the cochlea. The hair cells responding to higher frequency sounds are located closer to the basal end of the cochlea, and those most sensitive to lower frequency sounds are found toward the apical end of cochlea. The amount and the type of direct hair cell damage depends on the intensity of the sound. Exposure to noise at subtraumatic level exhibits a temporary shift in hearing sensitivity that returns to normal with time away from the hazardous exposure. However, higher sound levels damage the outer hair cells, stereocilia, further, including destruction of the intercilial bridges, and recovery takes longer. An even higher level of sound leads to a collapse of the stereocilia and the hair cell is eventually damaged permanently. If the outer hair cells are not functioning, a greater stimulation is required to initiate a nervous impulse; thus, the threshold sensitivity of inner hair cells is raised, which is perceived as a hearing loss. Once damaged, the auditory sensory cells cannot repair themselves nor can the medical procedures restore normal function.

Diagnosis of NIHL

Audiometry is a standard test to detect and evaluate hearing loss. Audiometry is used to determine the auditory threshold of an individual to pure tones of 250-8000 Hz and sound levels between 10 (the hearing threshold of intact ears) and 110 dB (maximal damage). The patient should not have been exposed to noise during the previous 16 h to eliminate the effects of a temporary threshold shift. Air conduction is measured by ear phones placed on the ears, while bone conduction is measured by placing a vibrator in contact with the skull behind the ears. Each ear is evaluated separately and test results are reported on a graph known as an audiogram. Comparison of air and bone conduction allows classification of hearing loss as conductive or sensorineural. The audiogram in case of NIHL is characterized by an onset of hearing loss at 4000 Hz, visible as a dip in the audiogram. As exposure to excessive noise level continues, neighboring frequencies are progressively affected and the dip broadens, intruding into neighboring frequencies. NIHL is usually bilateral and shows a similar pattern in both the ears. The difference between the two ears should not exceed 15 dB at 500, 1000 and 2000 Hz and 30 dB at 3000, 4000 and 6000 Hz, respectively.

Grading of the Hearing Impairment

The WHO recommended the following classification on the basis of the pure tone audiogram taking the average of the thresholds of hearing for frequencies of 500, 1000, 2000 and 4000 Hz. Table shows the grading of hearing impairment.

Table: Grading of the hearing impairment

Grade of impairment	Corresponding audiometric ISO value	Performance	Recommendations
0 - No impairment	25 dB or better (better ear)	No or very slight hearing problems. Able to hear whispers	

1 - Slight impairment	26-40 dB (better ear)	Able to hear and repeat words spoken in normal voice at 1 m	Counseling. Hearing aids may be needed
2 - Moderate impairment	41-60 dB (better ear)	Able to hear and repeat words spoken in a raised voice at 1 m	Hearing aids usually recommended
3 - Severe impairment	61-80 dB (better ear)	Able to hear some words when shouted into the better ear	Hearing aids needed. If no hearing aids available, lipreading and signing should be taught
4 - Profound impairment including deafness	81 dB or greater (better ear)	Unable to hear and understand even a shouted voice	Hearing aids may help understand words. Additional rehabilitation needed. Lipreading and sometimes signing essential

Grades 2, 3 and 4 are classified as disabling hearing impairment. The audiometric ISO values are averages of values at 500, 1000, 2000 and 4000 Hz.

Calculation of the Hearing Impairment

To express the hearing impairment in terms of percentage, different countries and professional bodies have adopted their own system to calculate the percentage. One of the methods to find hearing impairment is as follows:

1. From the audiogram, calculate the average of the thresholds of hearing for frequencies of 500, 1000, 2000, 4000 and 6000 Hz.
2. Deduct from it 25 dB (as there is no impairment up to 25 dB).
3. Multiply it by 1.5.

This is the percentage of hearing impairment for that ear. Similarly, calculate the percentage of hearing impairment for the other ear. The percentage handicap of an individual is calculated using the formula given below.

$$\text{Percentage handicap of an individual} = \frac{(\text{Better ear}\,\% \times 5) + (\text{worse ear}\,\%)}{6}$$

Occupational NIHL

In a cross-sectional study, the hearing status of tractor-driving farmers (TDFs) was compared with that of non-TDFs. All participants were interviewed for details of work routine and noise exposures. Audiogram analysis showed higher prevalence of abnormalities in TDFs. TDFs more often had a higher frequency of hearing loss when compared with non-TDFs.

A study was conducted in heavy engineering industry, which included machines shop and press divisions. The sound levels ranged from 83 to 116 dBA. Hearing impairment was progressive in all the study groups.

In a textile mill weavers study, the sound levels were around 102-104 dBA and the hearing acuity of the textile weavers was found to be poor. NIHL at 4000 Hz was as high as 30 dB in the age range 25-29 years, 40 dB in the age range 30-34 years and 45 dB in the age range 35-39 years.

A study was conducted in a drug and pharmaceutical company where the noise levels were 100-105 dBA. Significant NIHL was found in the workers.

A survey on the effects of noise pollution on traffic policemen in the city of Hyderabad, India, carried out by the Society to Aid the Hearing Impaired, revealed that 76% had NIHL. Among these, all those who had completed 5 years in the traffic wing had hearing loss in various degrees.

The National institute of miners' health (NIMH) has carried out NIHL studies in various mines. NIHL was prevalent among 12.8% of the employees. Moderate NIHL was detected in 10.2% and severe NIHL was observed in 2.6% of the employees.

There are other industries like construction, printing, saw mills and crushers where the workers are exposed to high levels of noise throughout their lifetime of work. Studies regarding NIHL among the workers of these industries are not available.

Ear Protection and Conservation

The most effective way to prevent NIHL is to protect the worker from hazardous noise at the workplace. Hearing protectors should be used when engineering controls and work practices are not feasible for reducing noise exposure to safe levels. A personal hearing protection device is a device designed to reduce the level of sound reaching the eardrum. Ear muffs, ear plugs and ear canal caps are the main types of hearing protectors. To select hearing protectors, we should consider the following:

- The workers who will be wearing them.
- The need for compatibility with other safety equipment.
- Workplace conditions such as temperature, humidity and atmospheric pressure.

A variety of style should be provided so that workers may select a hearing protector on the basis of comfort, ease of use and handling and impact on communication. Each worker should receive individual training in the selection, fitting, use, repair and replacement of hearing protectors. The most common excuses reported by workers for not wearing hearing protectors include discomfort, interference with hearing speech and warning signals and the belief of workers that there is no control over an inevitable process that causes hearing loss. Given adequate education and training, workers can realize the crucial importance of wearing hearing protectors.

Ménière's Disease

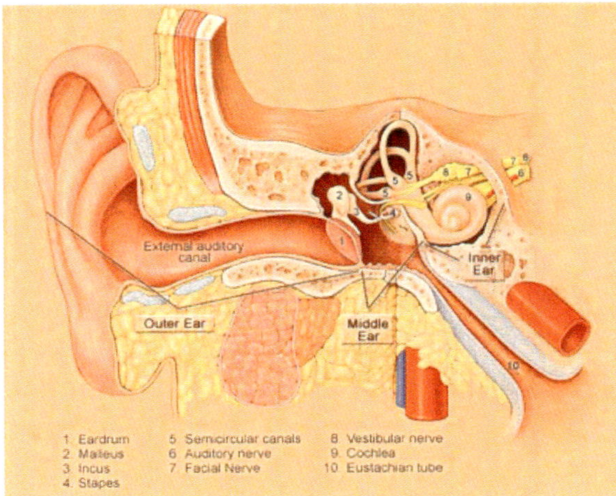

Figure: Normal inner ear.

In 1861, the French physician Prosper Meniere described a condition which now bears his name. Meniere's disease is a disorder of the inner ear that causes episodes of vertigo, ringing in the ears (tinnitus), a feeling of fullness or pressure in the ear, and fluctuating hearing loss. In figure, the area of the ear affected is the entire labyrinth, which includes both the semicircular canals and the cochlea.

Symptoms of Meniere's Disease

A typical attack of Meniere's disease is preceded by fullness in one ear. Hearing fluctuation or changes in tinnitus may also precede an attack. A Meniere's episode generally involves severe vertigo (spinning), imbalance, nausea and vomiting. The average attack lasts two to four hours. Following a severe attack, most people find that they are exhausted and must sleep for several hours. There is a large amount of variability in the duration of symptoms. Some people experience brief "shocks," and others have constant unsteadiness. The majority of people with Meniere's disease are over 40 years of age, with equal distribution between males and females.

A particularly disabling symptom is a sudden fall that may occur without warning. These are called otolithic crisis of Tumarkin, from the original description of Tumarkin (1936). These are attributed to sudden mechanical deformation of the otolith organs (utricle and saccule), causing a sudden activation of vestibular reflexes. Patients suddenly feel that they are tilted or falling (although they may be straight), and bring about much of the rapid repositioning themselves. This is a very disabling symptom as it occurs without warning and can result in severe injury. Often destructive treatment (for example labyrinthectomy or vestibular nerve section) is the only way to manage this problem. for more information about drop attacks.

Meniere's episodes may occur in clusters; that is, several attacks may occur within a short period of time. However, years may pass between episodes. Between the acute attacks, most people are free of symptoms or note mild imbalance and tinnitus.

Meniere's disease usually starts confined to one ear but it often extends to involve both ears over time so that after 30 years, 50% of patients with Meniere's have bilateral disease (Stahle et al, 1991). There is some controversy about this statistic however; some researchers suggest that the prevalence of bilaterality is as low as 17% (Silverstein, 1992). We suspect that this lower statistic is due to a lower duration of follow-up and that the 50% figure is more likely to be correct. Other possibilities, however, are selection bias and different patterns of the disease in different countries. Silverstein suggested that 75% of persons destined to become bilateral do so within five years.

In most cases, a progressive hearing loss occurs in the affected ear(s). A low-frequency sensorineural pattern is commonly found initially, but as time goes on, it usually changes into either a flat loss or a peaked pattern (click here for more information about hearing testing). Although an acute attack can be incapacitating, the disease itself is not fatal.

Migraines occur more frequently in patients with Meniere's disease. Meniere's patients who have associated migraines are reported to have an earlier age of disease onset and a higher rate of family history, suggesting a genetic component.

Meniere's disease affects roughly 0.2% of the population. Interestingly, the Framingham study found that 2% of the population of the United States believe they have Meniere's disease, suggesting that there is considerable chance of misdiagnosis.

Causes of Meniere's Disease

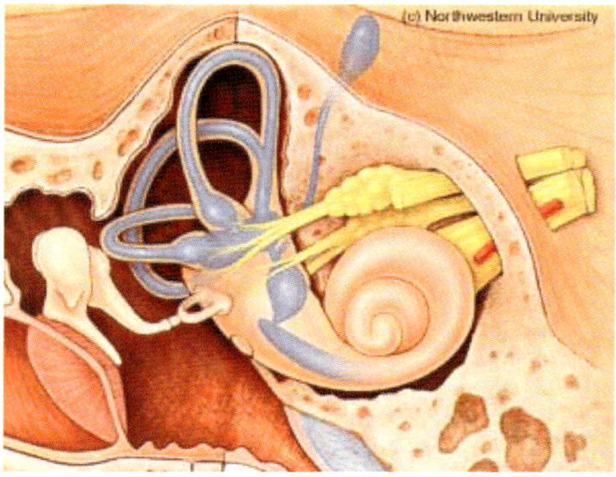

Figure: Normal membranous labyrinth

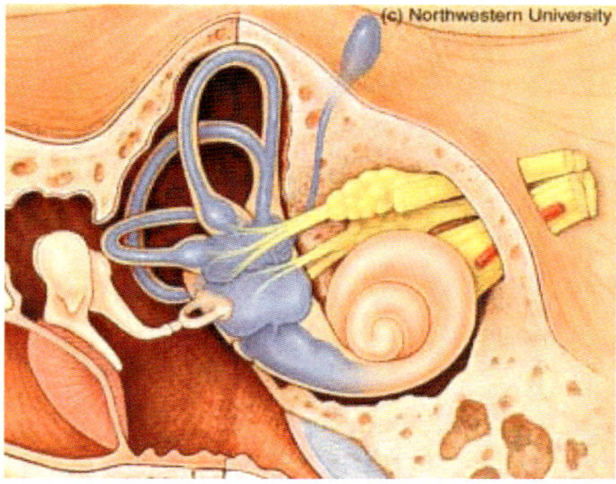

Dilated membranous labyrinth in Meniere's disease (Hydrops)

An acute attack of Meniere's disease is generally believed to result from fluctuating pressure of the fluid within the inner ear. This is called "hydrops". A system of membranes, called the membranous labyrinth, contains a fluid called endolymph. The membranes can become dilated like a balloon when pressure increases. One way for this to happen is when the drainage system, called the endolymphatic duct or sac is blocked. In some cases, the endolymphatic duct may be obstructed by scar tissue, or may be narrow from birth. In some cases there may be too much fluid secreted by the stria vascularis. Recently, some have pointed out that this "central hypothesis" of Meniere's is questionable, as many normal people without Meniere's have evidence of increased pressure in the inner ear too.

Abnormally enlarged fluid pathways into the ear, such as the vestibular aqueduct or cochlear aqueduct, may also be associated with Meniere's-like symptoms, but recent evidence is against a relationship between the cochlear aqueduct and Meniere's disease. In a review of literature, Ciuman (2009) stated that the endolymphatic sac in those with enlarged vestibular aqueduct was thin, whereas it was fibrous in those with Meniere's.

For the most part, the underlying cause of Meniere's disease is unknown. It is most often attributed to viral infections of the inner ear, head injury, a hereditary predisposition, and allergy.

Meniere's disease can cause hair cell death, as well as mechanical changes to the ear.

Hair Cell Death

The periodic admixture of perilymph and endolymph often kills hair cells in the inner ear. This is a gradual process over years, but frequently resulting in unilateral functional deafness. Cochlear (hearing) hair cells are the most sensitive. Vestibular (motion sensing) hair cells seem more resilient but there is also a slow decline in the caloric response in the diseased ear over roughly 15 years.

Mechanical Changes

Mechanical disruption of the inner ear is also likely, with dilation of the utricle and saccule of the ear being a well-known pathological finding. The saccule may dilate so that, in later stages, it is adherent to the underside of the stapes footplate. This mechanical disruption and distortion of normal inner ear structures may result in the gradual onset of a chronic unsteadiness, even when patients are not having attacks. The periodic dilation and shrinkage of the utricle is also a reasonable explanation for periodic attacks of another inner ear disorder, BPPV. Finally, it also seems likely that there may be a rupture of the suspensory system for the membranous labyrinth. This might create some mechanical instability of the utricle and saccule and consequently some chronic unsteadiness.

There is presently no evidence that Meniere's disease kills the cochleovestibular nerve (Kitamura et al, 1997). Although a recent study showed significant neural deterioration in a guinea pig model of endolymphatic hydrops, a hallmark of Meniere's.

Diagnosis of Meniere's Disease

Diagnosis is based on a combination of the right set of symptoms (usually episodic dizziness and hearing disturbance); hearing tests, which document that hearing is reduced after an attack, and then gets better; and exclusion of alternative causes. The differential diagnosis is broad and includes perilymph fistula, recurrent labyrinthitis, migraine, congenital ear malformations of many kinds, syphilis, tumors, Multiple Sclerosis, etc. The process of diagnosis usually includes hearing testing (audiometry), an ENG test, several blood tests (ANA, FTA), and an MRI scan of the head. Electrocochleography (ECOG) is helpful in difficult cases.

Hearing tests often begin with showing a fluctuating low-frequency sensorineural hearing loss. Over years, this gradually progresses to a "peaked" pattern with both low- and high-tone reduction, and finally a "flat" pattern, typically 50 db loss (110 db would be completely deaf). While some people have hearing that fluctuates like this without any further symptoms of dizziness or tinnitus, in most cases, this does not progress to Meniere's disease (Schaaf et al, 2001). A recent study examined the relationship between hearing fluctuation and vertigo attacks (Neill et al., 2010). The studies concluded that hearing fluctuation often occurs independently of vertiginous episodes.

Ménière's Disease Treatment

At the present time there is no cure for Meniere's disease, but there are ways to manage the condition and help you control symptoms. Treatment for Meniere's disease falls into the following categories:

- Medication;
- Noninvasive pressure pulse generator (Meniett Device);
- Surgery;
- Diet.

Medications for an Acute Attack of Meniere's

Medications commonly used for an acute attack include the following:

- Meclizine (Antivert), chewable (Bonine). Dose ranges from 12.5 twice a day to 50 mg three times a day.
- Lorazepam (Ativan) 0.5 mg. Usual dose is twice a day. This medication can be taken under the tongue.
- Phenergan (orally or suppository). Usual dose is 12.5 mg every 12 hours as needed for vomiting.

- Compazine (orally or suppository). Usual dose is 5 mg every 12 hours as needed for vomiting.
- Dexamethasone (Decadron) 4 mg orally for 4 days.

Medications used between Attacks

1. Diuretics:
    - Dyazide (Triamterine/HCTZ)
2. Vestibular Suppressants:
    - Klonapin 0.5 mg twice a day or as needed;
    - Lorazepam (Ativan) 0.5 mg twice a day or as needed;
    - Diazepam (Valium) 2 mg twice a day or as needed;
    - Meclizine (Antivert) 12.5 mg to 25 mg as needed up to 3- to 4-times a day.
3. Calcium Channel Blockers:
    - Verapamil (Calan is one brand name);
    - Flunarizine/Cinnarizine (not available in the USA);
    - Nimodipine (Nimotop — generally too expensive to be practical).
4. Steroids (Rarely Used):
    - Dexamethasone (note that intratympanic administration is controversial);
    - Prednisone.
5. Immune Suppressants:
    - Methotrexate;
    - Steroids;
    - Embrel.
6. Agents that are Controversial:
    - Serc (beta-histine);
    - Histamine injections;
    - Homeopathic treatments, such as VertigoHeel;
    - Antiviral therapy (such as Acyclovir);
    - Intratympanic dexamethasone.

Way to Manage an Attack of Meniere's Disease

During an acute attack, lay down on a firm surface. Stay as motionless as possible, with your eyes open and fixed on a stationary object. Do not try to drink or sip water, as you would be very likely to vomit. Stay like this until the severe vertigo (spinning) passes, then get up SLOWLY. After the attack subsides, you will probably feel very tired and need to sleep for several hours.

If vomiting persists and you are unable to take fluids for longer than 24 hours (12 hours for children), contact your doctor. He or she can prescribe nausea medication, and/or vestibular suppressant medication. Your doctor may wish to see you. Antivert and Ativan are commonly used vestibular suppressant medications and Compazine or Phenergan are commonly used medications for nausea.

Precaution of Meniere's Disease

Between attacks, medication may be prescribed to help regulate the fluid pressure in your inner ear, thereby reducing the severity and frequency of the Meniere's episodes. Dyazide is the most common medication for this purpose. Neptazine can be used when response to Dyazide isn't good enough. Verapamil (typical dose: 120 SR) sometimes reduces the frequency of attacks. Some physicians prescribe Histamine injections. Prednisone or other steroids (for example Decadron) are occasionally helpful in short bursts. Vestibular suppressants such as Antivert (meclizine) or Klonazepam are used on an as-needed basis.

There are a number of new medications that do not have much of a track record that can be tried under the supervision of your doctor. There also some unusual medications which are either considered "alternative" or which are available only outside the United States which might be worth considering.

The hydrops diet regimen will probably be recommended. This is an important part of treatment for virtually all patients with Meniere's disease. Experience has shown that STRICT adherence to this dietary regimen will result in significant improvement in most patients.

The purpose of treatment between attacks is to prevent or reduce the number of episodes, and to decrease the chances of further hearing loss. A permanent tinnitus (ringing in the ears) or a progressive hearing loss may be the consequence of long-term Meniere's disease. Hearing aids may be necessary.

Noninvasive Pressure Pulse Generator (Meniett Device)

The Meniett device, manufactured by Medtronic (R), is a noninvasive treatment option that works by sending small pulses of pressure into the ear canal. It is thought that this reduces symptoms of Meniere's disease by eliminating excess endolymphatic fluid within the ear. The Meniett device is used at home, typically three times per day, five minutes at a time. Researchers have reported that the majority of patients (about 70 percent) report significant improvement in symptoms with the use of the Meniett device.

Surgery and Destructive Treatments of Meniere's Disease

In extremely severe cases, treatments that deaden the inner ear such as gentamicin injections or surgery may be considered. This is a last resort for persons who have severe attacks which are disabling. At present, we favor gentamicin for most instances where destructive treatments are being considered. Injections of gentamicin are given through the ear drum, through a small hole or through a small tube. This procedure allows the doctor to treat one side alone, without affecting the other. Typically, about four injections are given over a period of one month. Some researchers have reported improvements in 60 to 90 percent of patients with gentamicin, and Chung reported equally effective results with a single injection compared to multiple injections . Dizziness may reoccur one year later, requiring another series. Gentamicin injection can also result in hearing loss.

Although intratympanic steroids injections have also been recently used to treat Meniere's disease by Shea, the present consensus is that treatment has not yet been clearly proven to be effective or to have a reasonable scientific basis. Some studies suggest that it is no better than placebo.

Alternatively, a surgical treatment is used in which the vestibular nerve is clipped. This operation, called a vestibular neurectomy or vestibular nerve section is very effective in eliminating vertigo . While very effective, this procedure, especially the hearing-sparing variant, is presently generally felt to be of much higher risk than gentamicin injection. We presently do not recommend vestibular nerve section for Meniere's disease, except in situations where gentamicin injection has failed.

Another operation, called a labyrinthectomy, is recommended in persons who have lost all usable hearing or in whom vestibular nerve section is considered too dangerous. Again, this procedure seems most applicable to situations where gentamicin has failed.

A third operation, the endolymphatic shunt procedure, is used by some doctors to relieve pressure in the inner ear (Derebery et al., 2010; Brinson, 2007). Unfortunately, while the shunt would seem to be a logical thing to do, in most studies, the shunt procedure does not appear to be better than doing nothing (Silverstein and Rosenberg, 1992). This may be because the shunt can easily get plugged up. One recent study did conclude a higher success rate than gentamicin injection (Derebery et al., 2010). We do not presently recommend this procedure for our patients except in unusual situations. A recent trend is to make an attempt to damage the sac, in addition to improving its drainage. As the sac is the immune organ of the ear, this idea makes sense if one is attempting to immunosuppress the ear.

For bilateral Meniere's disease, when the patient is incapacitated and it cannot be determined which ear is causing the dizziness, intramuscular streptomycin (1 gm twice a day) can be given on an outpatient basis until the first sign of ototoxicity develops. This treatment can generally reduce or eliminate vertigo spells without affecting hearing. This treatment however damages the inner ear and causes bilateral vestibular paresis, which has its own set of symptoms and disability.

Hydrops Diet

The fluid-filled hearing and balance structures of the inner ear normally function independent of the body's overall fluid/blood system. In a normal inner ear, the fluid is maintained at a constant volume and contains specific concentrations of sodium, potassium, chloride and other electrolytes. This fluid bathes the sensory cells of the inner ear and allows them to function normally.

With injury or degeneration of the inner ear structures, independent control is lost, and the volume and concentration of the inner ear fluid fluctuates with changes in the body's fluid/blood. This fluctuation causes the symptoms of hydrops (pressure or fullness in the ears), tinnitus (ringing in the ears), hearing loss, dizziness and imbalance.

Tinnitus

Tinnitus (TIN-ih-tus) is the perception of noise or ringing in the ears. A common problem, tinnitus affects about 1 in 5 people. Tinnitus isn't a condition itself — it's a symptom of an underlying condition, such as age-related hearing loss, ear injury or a circulatory system disorder.

Although bothersome, tinnitus usually isn't a sign of something serious. Although it can worsen with age, for many people, tinnitus can improve with treatment. Treating an identified underlying cause sometimes helps. Other treatments reduce or mask the noise, making tinnitus less noticeable.

Symptoms

Tinnitus involves the annoying sensation of hearing sound when no external sound is present. Tinnitus symptoms include these types of phantom noises in your ears:

- Ringing
- Buzzing
- Roaring

- Clicking
- Hissing

The phantom noise may vary in pitch from a low roar to a high squeal, and you may hear it in one or both ears. In some cases, the sound can be so loud it can interfere with your ability to concentrate or hear actual sound. Tinnitus may be present all the time, or it may come and go.

There are two kinds of tinnitus:

- Subjective tinnitus is tinnitus only you can hear. This is the most common type of tinnitus. It can be caused by ear problems in your outer, middle or inner ear. It also can be caused by problems with the hearing (auditory) nerves or the part of your brain that interprets nerve signals as sound (auditory pathways).
- Objective tinnitus is tinnitus your doctor can hear when he or she does an examination. This rare type of tinnitus may be caused by a blood vessel problem, a middle ear bone condition or muscle contractions.

Causes

A number of health conditions can cause or worsen tinnitus. In many cases, an exact cause is never found.

A common cause of tinnitus is inner ear cell damage. Tiny, delicate hairs in your inner ear move in relation to the pressure of sound waves. This triggers ear cells to release an electrical signal through a nerve from your ear (auditory nerve) to your brain. Your brain interprets these signals as sound. If the hairs inside your inner ear are bent or broken, they can "leak" random electrical impulses to your brain, causing tinnitus.

Other causes of tinnitus include other ear problems, chronic health conditions, and injuries or conditions that affect the nerves in your ear or the hearing center in your brain.

Common Causes of Tinnitus

In many people, tinnitus is caused by one of these conditions:

- Age-related hearing loss - For many people, hearing worsens with age, usually starting around age 60. Hearing loss can cause tinnitus. The medical term for this type of hearing loss is presbycusis.
- Exposure to loud noise - Loud noises, such as those from heavy equipment, chain saws and firearms, are common sources of noise-related hearing loss. Portable music devices, such as MP3 players or iPods, also can cause noise-related

hearing loss if played loudly for long periods. Tinnitus caused by short-term exposure, such as attending a loud concert, usually goes away; long-term exposure to loud sound can cause permanent damage.

- Earwax blockage - Earwax protects your ear canal by trapping dirt and slowing the growth of bacteria. When too much earwax accumulates, it becomes too hard to wash away naturally, causing hearing loss or irritation of the eardrum, which can lead to tinnitus.
- Ear bone changes - Stiffening of the bones in your middle ear (otosclerosis) may affect your hearing and cause tinnitus. This condition, caused by abnormal bone growth, tends to run in families.

Other Causes of Tinnitus

Some causes of tinnitus are less common, including:

- Meniere's disease - Tinnitus can be an early indicator of Meniere's disease, an inner ear disorder that may be caused by abnormal inner ear fluid pressure.
- TMJ disorders - Problems with the temporomandibular joint, the joint on each side of your head in front of your ears, where your lower jawbone meets your skull, can cause tinnitus.
- Head injuries or neck injuries - Head or neck trauma can affect the inner ear, hearing nerves or brain function linked to hearing. Such injuries generally cause tinnitus in only one ear.
- Acoustic neuroma - This noncancerous (benign) tumor develops on the cranial nerve that runs from your brain to your inner ear and controls balance and hearing. Also called vestibular schwannoma, this condition generally causes tinnitus in only one ear.

Blood Vessel Disorders Linked to Tinnitus

In rare cases, tinnitus is caused by a blood vessel disorder. This type of tinnitus is called pulsatile tinnitus. Causes include:

- Atherosclerosis - With age and buildup of cholesterol and other deposits, major blood vessels close to your middle and inner ear lose some of their elasticity — the ability to flex or expand slightly with each heartbeat. That causes blood flow to become more forceful, making it easier for your ear to detect the beats. You can generally hear this type of tinnitus in both ears.
- Head and neck tumors - A tumor that presses on blood vessels in your head or neck (vascular neoplasm) can cause tinnitus and other symptoms.

- High blood pressure - Hypertension and factors that increase blood pressure, such as stress, alcohol and caffeine, can make tinnitus more noticeable.
- Turbulent blood flow - Narrowing or kinking in a neck artery (carotid artery) or vein in your neck (jugular vein) can cause turbulent, irregular blood flow, leading to tinnitus.
- Malformation of capillaries - A condition called arteriovenous malformation (AVM), abnormal connections between arteries and veins, can result in tinnitus. This type of tinnitus generally occurs in only one ear.

Medications that Cause Tinnitus

A number of medications may cause or worsen tinnitus. Generally, the higher the dose of these medications, the worse tinnitus becomes. Often the unwanted noise disappears when you stop using these drugs. Medications known to cause or worsen tinnitus include:

- Antibiotics, including polymyxin B, erythromycin, vancomycin and neomycin;
- Cancer medications, including mechlorethamine and vincristine;
- Water pills (diuretics), such as bumetanide, ethacrynic acid or furosemide;
- Quinine medications used for malaria or other health conditions;
- Certain antidepressants may worsen tinnitus;
- Aspirin taken in uncommonly high doses (usually 12 or more a day).

Risk Factors

Anyone can experience tinnitus, but these factors may increase your risk:

- Loud noise exposure - Prolonged exposure to loud noise can damage the tiny sensory hair cells in your ear that transmit sound to your brain. People who work in noisy environments — such as factory and construction workers, musicians, and soldiers — are particularly at risk.
- Age - As you age, the number of functioning nerve fibers in your ears declines, possibly causing hearing problems often associated with tinnitus.
- Gender - Men are more likely to experience tinnitus.
- Smoking - Smokers have a higher risk of developing tinnitus.
- Cardiovascular problems - Conditions that affect your blood flow, such as high blood pressure or narrowed arteries (atherosclerosis), can increase your risk of tinnitus.

Complications

Tinnitus can significantly affect quality of life. Although it affects people differently, if you have tinnitus, you also may experience:

- Fatigue
- Stress
- Sleep problems
- Trouble concentrating
- Memory problems
- Depression
- Anxiety and irritability

Treating these linked conditions may not affect tinnitus directly, but it can help you feel better.

Prevention

In many cases, tinnitus is the result of something that can't be prevented. However, some precautions can help prevent certain kinds of tinnitus.

- Use hearing protection - Over time, exposure to loud noise can damage the nerves in the ears, causing hearing loss and tinnitus. If you use chain saws, are a musician, work in an industry that uses loud machinery or use firearms (especially pistols or shotguns), always wear over-the-ear hearing protection.
- Turn down the volume - Long-term exposure to amplified music with no ear protection or listening to music at very high volume through headphones can cause hearing loss and tinnitus.
- Take care of your cardiovascular health - Regular exercise, eating right and taking other steps to keep your blood vessels healthy can help prevent tinnitus linked to blood vessel disorders.

Tinnitus Treatment

The first step is to treat any underlying cause of tinnitus.

This may involve:

- Prompt care for an ear infection.
- Discontinuing any ototoxic medications.

- Treating any temporomandibular joint (TMJ) problems, which affect the joint between the jaw bone and the cheek bone.

There is no cure for most cases of tinnitus. Most people become accustomed to it and learn to tune it out. Ignoring it rather than focusing on it can provide relief.

When this does not work, the individual may benefit from treatment for the effects of tinnitus, insomnia, anxiety, hearing difficulties, social isolation, and depression. Dealing with these issues can significantly improve a person's quality of life.

Home Remedies

Here are some other things a person can do to manage tinnitus and its effects.

Sound therapy uses external noise to mask the individual's perception of tinnitus. Low-level background music, white noise, or specialized ear maskers can help.

The choice of sound should be pleasant to the individual. Masking devices offer temporary relief, and the awareness of tinnitus returns when the sound therapy is turned off.

Hearing aids are a common type of sound therapy. They amplify environmental sounds and redirect attention to those noises instead of the tinnitus.

Tinnitus retraining therapy (TRT) involves retraining the auditory system to accept the abnormal sounds of tinnitus as natural rather than disruptive.

It involves help from a trained professional and wearing a device that emits low-level white noise. Ongoing counseling sessions can help people cope with the tinnitus.

This therapy's success is proportionate to the severity of the tinnitus and the individual's overall mental health.

Follow-up studies suggest that TRT provides relief for around 80 percent of people with tinnitus.

Cognitive behavioral therapy (CBT) can help relieve depression in people with tinnitus, although it does not appear to reduce the sound.

Healthy Lifestyle

One way to prevent tinnitus, and possibly hearing loss, is by avoiding exposure to loud noises.

To prevent hearing damage from developing or worsening:

- Use hearing protection, such as ear mufflers and earplugs, in noisy environments;
- Play personal listening devices at a moderate volume.

Improving wellness will not stop tinnitus, but overall wellbeing can help limit its intensity and provide physical and emotional benefits.

Exercise, healthy eating, good sleeping habits, avoiding smoking and excessive alcohol, recreational and social activities, and stress management and relaxation techniques can all help achieve optimum wellness.

Unfortunately, once the damage is done, there is no way to reverse it.

Hyperacusis

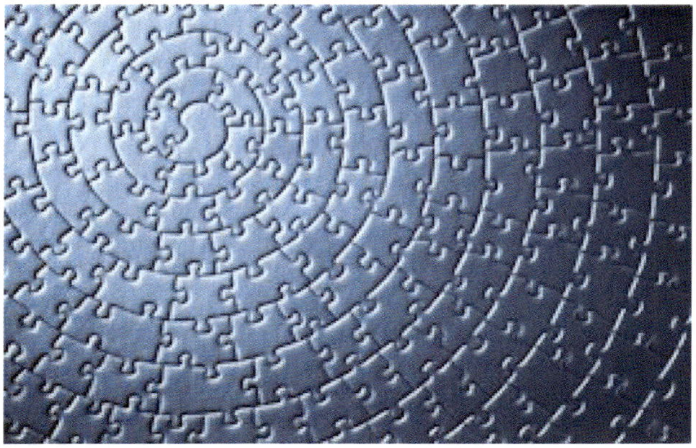

Imagine being at a movie where the sound track is turned to the highest volume. Actors' voices are screaming at you. After five minutes, you leave holding your ears and cursing the theater for its poor judgment. Turning newspaper pages, running water in the kitchen sink, your child placing dishes and silverware on the table - all are intolerable to your ears. A baby cries or a truck screeches its brakes to a halt and the sound is excruciating.

The person who has hyperacusis can't simply get up and walk away from noise. Instead, the volume on the whole world seems stuck on high. Hyperacusis is defined as a collapsed tolerance to normal environmental sounds. Ears also lose most of their dynamic range.

Dynamic range is the ability of the ear to deal with quick shifts in sound loudness. Suddenly everyday noises sound unbearably or painfully loud. The disorder is often chronic and usually accompanied by tinnitus (ringing in the ears), but can occur in patients who have little or no measurable hearing loss.

Hyperacusis differs from recruitment, which is an abnormal growth in the perception of loudness accompanied with hearing loss. With recruitment, loud noises are uncomfortable. With hyperacusis, all sounds are too loud.

Most patients also experience inner ear pain or a feeling of fullness (pressure) in the ears. This pressure in the ears can best be described as the feeling one normally gets when descending in an airplane. Hyperacusis can be devastating to the patient's career, relationships, and peace of mind. Finding the proper diagnosis is difficult because few doctors understand hyperacusis.

A Life Altering Condition

Hyperacusis makes living in this noisy world difficult and dramatically changes the patient's pattern of life. Moving about, traveling, and communicating with others is challenging. Ear protection must be worn in areas that seem too loud. This includes earplugs, industrial earmuffs or both if necessary.

Even then, many vocational and recreational activities must be curtailed or eliminated because, although protection reduces the noise entering the ears, it sometimes seems insufficient to block out certain frequencies or noise intensities. The things most of us take for granted, such as driving a car, walking down the street, riding a bicycle, listening to the TV, stereo, someone speaking over a telephone or microphone, shopping, attending indoor events, dining at restaurants, taking vacations, or participating in group activities often are difficult or impossible. Many have difficulty using a vacuum cleaner, a hammer, a lawn mower, power tools, ride a motor boat or motorcycle.

Most jobs involve some level of noise. In some cases, the patient may need to seek other employment or attempt to secure disability with the help of an understanding doctor. Loud noise exposure generally makes the condition worse and exacerbates the accompanying tinnitus. Patients report they perceive sound - even their own voice - as uncomfortably loud and this not only causes tinnitus to increase but may also cause inner ear discomfort or a popping reflex in the ear. In fact some patients actually try to change the pitch of their own voice to accomodate their ears. This may help their ears but a patient can become hoarse in the process.

In cases not involving aural trauma to the inner ear, hyperacusis can also be acquired as a result of damage to the brain or the neurological system. In these cases, hyperacusis can be defined as a cerebral processing problem specific to how the brain perceives sound. In rare cases, hyperacusis may be caused by a vestibular disorder. This type of hyperacusis, called vestibular hyperacusis, is caused by the brain perceiving certain sounds as motion input as well as auditory input. In some cases, vestibular hyperacusis can affect the autonomic system and cause problems such as loss of consciousness, mental confusion, nausea, or extreme fatigue.

Causes of Hyperacusis

Some first develop hyperacusis in one ear, but in most cases both ears ultimately become affected. Hyperacusis can come on slowly or suddenly. Some patients say they developed hypersensitivity to sound over a period of time. Others may come down with hyperacusis suddenly by attending a rock concert, firing a gun, air bag deployment in their car, fireworks or any extremely loud sound.

Other causes may include job related noise exposure, drugs, Lyme's disease, Meniere's, Temporomandibular Joint Syndrome (TMJ), head injury, Superior Canal Dehiscence Syndrome (SCDS), postoperative surgery, autism or Down Syndrome.

The appearance of hyperacusis in some of these disorders may provide clues as to the cause of hyperacusis. Sometimes it disappears once the patient heals from the surgery, Meniere's goes into remission, or TMJ is resolved.

The protective mechanisms a normal ear employs to minimize the harmful effects of loud noise are malfunctioning, so noise may seem too loud even with hearing protection. There is some speculation that the efferent portion of the auditory nerve has been affected - efferent meaning fibers that originate in the brain, which serve to regulate incoming sounds. This theory about hyperacusis suggests that the efferent fibers of the auditory nerve are selectively damaged while the hair cells that allow us to hear pure tones in an audiometric evaluation remain intact. Some have said that it involves a direct malfunction of the facial nerve; as a result, the stapedius muscle is unable to dampen sound.

Since an estimated 10% of all tinnitus patients have no measurable hearing impairment; it comes as no surprise that other ear pathologies including hyperacusis can occur in the absence of hearing loss. Others feel hyperacusis is purely a central processing problem limited to how the brain perceives sound. Hyperacusis is not uncommon. It has been said that 5 million patients have tinnitus and 40% of those patients have hearing sensitivity or hyperacusis. Drug companies in our world today are especially interested in finding drugs that help large groups of people. This is very profitable for them. From that standpoint alone, research is being done to solve tinnitus. Some dominant voices in the world of tinnitus have said that tinnitus and hyperacusis are two sides of the same coin. If a cure is found for one, it is likely that a cure will be found for the other. In the meantime hyperacusis is a mystery but clues are beginning to surface which are very encouraging and hopeful.

Hyperacusis Treatment

If you suspect you have the condition, you'll want to see an otolaryngologist or an ear, nose and throat doctor (ENT). They'll look at your ears closely, note your medical history and confirm the condition through a hearing test.

Hearing tests typically record minus decibel levels and reveal normal hearing sensitivity. But, this doesn't indicate you hear better than other people when you have hyperacusis. Rather, it's a clear indication you have an issue with how your brain processes sound.

When there's a low tolerance to sound coupled with hearing loss, it's known as recruitment. This is where you can't hear soft sounds, but loud sounds are distorted or intolerable. For instance, with recruitment, you may have a below 50 decibels hearing loss, but still find noise over 80 decibels intolerable.

What's causing your hyperacusis is what will determine your hyperacusis treatment options. Sometimes, your sound sensitivity may improve by itself, such as with injuries to your ear or brain.

Sound Desensitization

If this isn't the case, your doctor may suggest sound desensitization where a specialist will work closely with you to help you how to cope with sound. Each day, they'll have you listen to extremely quiet sounds for a certain amount of time and then gradually build it up to louder sounds.

Usually, you'll wear a device on both ears or one affected ear. The noise typically sounds like static, therefore, it shouldn't cause you pain or bother you. It may take you up to a year to benefit fully from this therapy.

Not enough research has been done on other hyperacusis treatments like relaxation exercises or acupuncture to confirm they're useful and can help.

Auditory Integration Therapy (AIT)

AIT is usually used in treatment for autism and involves listening to different volumes of music for a certain amount of time each day.

Medication, while not always used as a treatment option, is also available to help manage hyperacusis-related stress.

You may be tempted to wear earplugs when you have hyperacusis or steer clear of social situations where there's potential for noise that can bother you. Doing these things can provide you with short-term relief, however, they can also worsen your symptoms over the long-term since after you finally go out in public or take your earplugs off, the noise seems louder.

Musical Ear Syndrome

Musical Ear Syndrome (MES), a term first coined in 2004 by Neil G. Bauman, Ph.D. refers to a condition in which those with hearing loss experience musical auditory hallucinations. According to Bauman, auditory hallucinations can range from simple sounds such as "ringing, roaring, buzzing, hissing, etc.," to complex sounds, such as music, singing and "voices that sound vaguely like a radio broadcast playing in another room." Those with MES tend to experience hearing sounds in the complex range. According to Bauman, the most commonly conjured tunes heard by more than half of people who experience MES are Christmas carols and patriotic music.

Auditory Hallucinations

These experiences are in fact auditory hallucinations, in which one experiences phantom sensory stimulation in the absence of real sensory stimuli. Of all the sensory hallucinations that humans can experience (sight, smell, taste, visual or feeling), auditory is the most common.

Auditory hallucinations are so common because of the very reason that Musical Ear Syndrome develops. It is a result of hearing loss, where the brain notices a lack of auditory stimulation and reacts by "filling in the blanks," or providing stimuli where there is none.

Hearing loss is the third most common chronic health condition in the United States. Moreover, it affects the elderly in more substantial percentages. Older folks with hearing loss tend to live quieter lives, in which auditory stimulation is sharply absent. Of course, another contributing factor may be certain types of medications, which are also disproportionately used by the aged.

Common, but Underreported

For fear of being deemed mad, Musical Ear Syndrome is a condition that is hugely underreported. One person suffering from Musical Ear Syndrome reports her fear of telling others of her experience, saying "I was afraid I was going nuts. I never said one word to anyone about the strange music I was hearing because I didn't want them to think I was crazy." However, it is also a common condition experienced by approximately 10% of those with hearing loss.

It's almost always directly linked to tinnitus, which is a ringing or buzzing sound heard but not present. This is a more culturally acceptable form of hearing phantom sounds, which is why the number of those afflicted might be more representative. Current data reports that 50 million Americans live with tinnitus.

There's a quick rule of thumb to rule out psychiatric auditory hallucinations and diagnose Musical Ear Syndrome: psychiatric hallucinations classically present as hearing voices. This means that a clear voice speaks to or about you and can be engaged in conversation. What's more, the topics or focus of the voice tend to be personally meaningful.

Comparatively, Musical Ear Syndrome sufferers tend to hear music or singing. If a spoken voice is heard, it is usually indistinct and vague.

Sound it Out

One way to alleviate the burden of Musical Ear Syndrome is to expose one's self to increased audio information. If your brain is dead set on providing you auditory sensory, then you might as well give it what it wants. That means turning up the radio or television, or better yet, socializing with others in conversation. This benefit is twofold as it attacks the silence and also gets the afflicted out of their isolating patterns. Reclusion in the elderly and particularly those with hearing loss is a powerful contributor to feelings of depression.

Speak with your doctor about your current medications if you think they might be a contributing factor in your auditory hallucinations. With their guidance, you can begin to eliminate obvious choices and pay attention to whether your Musical Ear Syndrome seems to be less present.

Be Mindful

Another and potentially more difficult way to treat Musical Ear Syndrome is by training the brain to ignore the phantom sounds. This could be as old school as wearing a rubber band around your wrist and snapping it when you begin to hear what isn't there. Immediately turn on the radio or another audio device and concentrate instead on real sounds that are present.

You might also take a new school approach and begin a meditation practice. Though thought of as new school, meditation is actually an ancient art practiced in many cultures for thousands of years. A steady practice results in more focused control of the brain and its thoughts, thereby teaching you strategies for ignoring the mind's grand productions.

Musical Ear Syndrome Treatment

The focus of treatment for the syndrome is to improve the hearing of the patient with hearing aids and to encourage them to enrich their environment with sound. That way, the brain isn't filling in the gaps with its own auditory hallucinations. If you are using any medications that might cause auditory hallucinations, your physician may change them or eliminate them. Some people may also benefit from anti-anxiety or anti-depressant medications.

References

- WHO (2008). The global burden of disease: 2004 update (PDF). Geneva, Switzerland: World Health Organization. p. 35. ISBN 9789241563710. Archived (PDF)from the original on 2013-06-24
- What-is-hyperacusis-definition-symptoms-causes-and-treatment-options: houstonent.com, Retrieved 30 June 2018

- Olusanya, BO; Neumann, KJ; Saunders, JE (1 May 2014). "The global burden of disabling hearing impairment: a call to action". Bulletin of the World Health Organization. 92 (5): 367–73. doi:10.2471/blt.13.128728. PMC 4007124. PMID 24839326
- Improve-your-hearing: starkey.com, Retrieved 23 May 2018
- "1.1 billion people at risk of hearing loss WHO highlights serious threat posed by exposure to recreational noise" (PDF). who.int. 27 February 2015. Archived (PDF) from the original on 1 May 2015. Retrieved 2 March 2015
- What-is-spatial-hearing-loss-and-how-is-it-treated: hearatlanta.com, Retrieved 3 July 2018
- Curhan, Sharon G.; Shargorodsky, Josef; Eavey, Roland; Curhan, Gary C. (2012-02-29). "Analgesic Use and the Risk of Hearing Loss in Women". Oxford Journals: American Journal of EPIDEMIOLOGY. Archived from the original on 2015-12-14
- Graham, edited by John M.; Baguley, David M. (2009). Ballantyne's Deafness (7th ed.). Chichester: John Wiley & Sons. p. 16. ISBN 978-0-470-74441-3.
- Causes-conductive-hearing-loss: audicus.com, Retrieved 30 June 2018
- Lasak, JM; Allen, P; McVay, T; Lewis, D (Mar 2014). "Hearing loss: diagnosis and management". Primary care. 41 (1): 19–31. doi:10.1016/j.pop.2013.10.003. PMID 24439878
- Goines, Lisa; Hagler, Louis (March 2007). "Noise Pollution: A Modern Plague". Southern Medical Journal. 100: 287–294. doi:10.1097/smj.0b013e3180318be5. Archived from the original on 8 September 2017. Retrieved 26 November 2014
- Common-causes-of-sensorineural-hearing-loss-50276: healthyhearing.com, Retrieved 29 June 2018
- World Health Organization, WHO (2017). Global costs of unaddressed hearing loss and cost-effectiveness of interventions: a WHO report. Geneva: World Health Organization. pp. 5–10. ISBN 978-92-4-151204-6

Permissions

All chapters in this book are published with permission under the Creative Commons Attribution Share Alike License or equivalent. Every chapter published in this book has been scrutinized by our experts. Their significance has been extensively debated. The topics covered herein carry significant information for a comprehensive understanding. They may even be implemented as practical applications or may be referred to as a beginning point for further studies.

We would like to thank the editorial team for lending their expertise to make the book truly unique. They have played a crucial role in the development of this book. Without their invaluable contributions this book wouldn't have been possible. They have made vital efforts to compile up to date information on the varied aspects of this subject to make this book a valuable addition to the collection of many professionals and students.

This book was conceptualized with the vision of imparting up-to-date and integrated information in this field. To ensure the same, a matchless editorial board was set up. Every individual on the board went through rigorous rounds of assessment to prove their worth. After which they invested a large part of their time researching and compiling the most relevant data for our readers.

The editorial board has been involved in producing this book since its inception. They have spent rigorous hours researching and exploring the diverse topics which have resulted in the successful publishing of this book. They have passed on their knowledge of decades through this book. To expedite this challenging task, the publisher supported the team at every step. A small team of assistant editors was also appointed to further simplify the editing procedure and attain best results for the readers.

Apart from the editorial board, the designing team has also invested a significant amount of their time in understanding the subject and creating the most relevant covers. They scrutinized every image to scout for the most suitable representation of the subject and create an appropriate cover for the book.

The publishing team has been an ardent support to the editorial, designing and production team. Their endless efforts to recruit the best for this project, has resulted in the accomplishment of this book. They are a veteran in the field of academics and their pool of knowledge is as vast as their experience in printing. Their expertise and guidance has proved useful at every step. Their uncompromising quality standards have made this book an exceptional effort. Their encouragement from time to time has been an inspiration for everyone.

The publisher and the editorial board hope that this book will prove to be a valuable piece of knowledge for students, practitioners and scholars across the globe.

Index

A

Absolute Threshold, 1, 32-33, 141

Acoustic Reflex, 30, 45-50, 91

Acoustics, 34, 134, 142, 193

Audiogram, 11-12, 96, 98, 100, 102, 152-153, 160, 163, 173, 178, 181, 201-202

Audiometer, 4, 92-93, 95, 100, 102, 123-124, 148, 151

Audiometry, 32, 91-95, 97-100, 102, 124, 148-149, 163, 173-174, 178, 183, 189-190, 201, 207

Auditory Canal, 38, 46, 181

Auditory Cortex, 3, 24, 36, 62, 66-68, 74, 76, 79, 84-87, 89, 103-106, 149, 159, 161

Auditory Hallucinations, 220-222

Auditory Scene Analysis, 91, 119-120, 123

Auditory Stimuli, 68, 88-89, 92, 99, 198

Autoimmune Disease, 94, 155-156

B

Bone Conduction, 5-7, 92, 97-98, 100, 169, 173, 201

Brain Stem, 35-36, 68

Bushy Cells, 72, 74-75, 77, 109

C

Cochlea, 3, 6-7, 13, 24-26, 36-37, 46-50, 53-58, 61-62, 65, 67, 69-71, 73-74, 76, 78, 80-82, 90, 94, 114-117, 156, 158, 162-163, 174-177, 179, 182, 196-197, 200, 204

Cochlear Damage, 113, 118, 156

Cochlear Implant, 112, 117, 168-169, 182

Corpus Callosum, 86, 195, 197-198

Critical Bandwidth, 25, 29

D

Deafness, 126, 150-151, 154-156, 162-164, 169, 174, 182-183, 186, 189, 202, 206, 223

Duplex Theory, 15-16, 18

E

Ear Canal, 2, 5, 13, 18-19, 36, 38-42, 46-47, 61, 94, 96, 99, 141, 158, 160, 162, 172, 184-185, 199, 203, 209, 213

Ear Protection, 165, 203, 215, 218

Eardrum, 3, 6-7, 18, 36, 39, 42-43, 64, 94, 158, 160, 162, 173, 187, 203, 213

Endolymph, 51-56, 58-59, 65-66, 205-206

Equal-loudness Contour, 138

F

Fletcher Munson Curve, 138

Frequency Weighting, 127, 129-130, 133

H

Headphone, 99

Hearing Aids, 1, 4-5, 11, 116-118, 150, 166, 168-169, 182, 185, 189, 194, 202, 209, 216, 222

Hearing Impairment, 5, 95, 113, 141, 150, 157, 161, 174, 181-182, 190, 199, 201-202, 219, 223

Hearing Loss, 1-2, 4-5, 7, 10-12, 26, 32, 46, 48-50, 81, 91-98, 101, 103, 112-119, 123, 129, 136, 141, 148, 150-166, 168-174, 177, 182-195, 197, 199-205, 207, 215-217, 219-223

Hearing Range, 1, 7-8, 10-11, 21, 60

Hearing Test, 11, 32, 91-92, 159-160, 173, 219

Human Auditory System, 14, 20-21, 23, 35, 106, 141

Hyperacusis, 4, 150, 217-220, 222

I

Inferior Colliculus, 14, 69, 71, 73, 76, 79, 83-84, 87

L

Lateral Lemniscus, 22, 69, 71-72, 75, 77, 83

Loudness, 8, 21-22, 31, 49, 62, 74, 106, 113, 120, 123, 126, 129, 138-139, 141, 143, 147, 185, 217

M

Masking, 1, 23-32, 91-92, 105-106, 108, 112, 114, 179, 216

Mastoid Air Cells, 43-45

Meniere's Disease, 4, 124, 204-207, 209-211, 213

Meningitis, 156, 164, 169, 172

Microphone, 42, 92, 125-129, 135-137, 168, 218

Middle Ear, 2-3, 13, 30, 36, 42-50, 53, 55, 61, 64-65, 81-82, 91-92, 94, 124, 141, 155-160, 162-163, 169, 172-173, 184-187, 191-192, 200, 212-213

Musical Ear Syndrome, 150, 220-222

Mutation, 154-155, 189

N

Noise Dosimeter, 127, 135-136

Noise Exposure, 117, 127, 134, 136, 138, 145, 152, 154-155, 164-165, 176, 199, 203, 214, 218-219

Noise Reduction, 117, 165
Noise-induced Hearing Loss, 5, 112, 115, 129, 153, 164-165, 171, 199-200

O
Octopus Cells, 70, 72-73
Outer Ear, 2, 19-20, 36-39, 42, 61, 63, 155, 158, 160, 184

P
Perilymph, 50-56, 58-59, 65-66, 155-156, 183, 206-207
Pinna, 2, 13-14, 18-21, 23, 36-38, 40, 63-64, 77, 99
Pitch, 8, 62, 91, 96, 106, 109, 111-112, 117-118, 120, 123, 139, 197, 212, 218
Pitch Perception, 109, 111-112, 117

S
Sensorineural Hearing Loss, 4, 48-49, 94-95, 97-98, 115, 150, 155-156, 160, 162-163, 170-174, 182-184, 207
Sequential Grouping, 120-121, 123
Signal Processing, 21, 116-117
Sound Exposure, 127, 131-132, 137
Sound Intensity, 62, 91, 96, 125-126, 138, 153-154, 200
Sound Level Meter, 91, 98, 125-128, 130, 132-136, 138
Sound Localization, 1, 12-16, 18-20, 22, 34, 74, 77, 109, 195
Spatial Hearing Loss, 194-195, 197
Speech Perception, 112, 114-116, 151
Stellate Cells, 70-75, 86
Superior Olivary Complex, 47, 69-72, 74-78, 83-84, 196
Superior Temporal Gyrus, 67, 85, 105
Sylvian Fissure, 85, 88

T
Temporal Bone, 38, 43, 45, 53
Temporal Envelope, 91, 103-104, 107, 111-113, 116, 118
Time Weighting, 127, 130-131
Tinnitus, 4, 32, 81, 114, 124, 150, 158, 183, 200, 204-205, 207, 209, 211-219, 221
Trapezoid Body, 69, 71-72, 75, 77-79, 84, 109

U
Unilateral Hearing Loss, 150, 164, 172, 190

V
Ventral Cochlear Nucleus, 47, 69-70, 72-76, 83, 109
Vestibule, 2-4, 50-53

W
Workplace Noise Regulation, 153, 165